# IN THE LOUPE

## The Secrets to Finding a Passion in Dentistry

Karl Walker-Finch

"Every day, think as you wake up, today I am fortunate to have woken up, I am alive, I have a precious human life, I am not going to waste it. I am going to use all my energies to develop myself and expand my heart out to others"

**The Dalai Lama**

# Contents

# Start Me Up
## The Rolling Stones

I don't think I'm being melodramatic (well, maybe a touch) to tell you that breaking my arm saved my life. It's November 2010, the patients are streaming in and out of my small surgery in a converted Wirral semi and I'm flying. I feel like I have a reasonable understanding of the NHS system even this early into my foundation year and I've overcome the initial stress of having to revise every night so I know what I'm doing for each procedure on tomorrow's list. It seems I've done a lot more work and I'm seeing a lot more patients than most of my fellow graduates and I'm fine with that, I want to be the best, the best should see the most patients, right? The more experienced dentists see more patients than me but I'm catching up, I'm winning the race to be the fastest and therefore the best, regardless of quality, I'm sure that'll come later.

I'm working with Lorraine, a wonderful, experienced dental nurse who's been working with newly qualified dentists for years. She's seen it all, she knows what you're good at and she knows when you need a little handholding through that tricky root canal treatment. She certainly knows dentistry a lot better than I do, though my arrogance means I don't realise this until much later.

Halfway through completing a large amalgam restoration (yes, there was a time when I still used amalgam) my stomach starts to cramp. The cramping crescendos until I have to step back from my patient to catch my breath. I'm incapable of doing or saying anything for the moment. It only lasts for about a minute but feels like an hour. I look around, I think I got away with it, the patient's still lying there, mouth wide open and Lorraine looks like she's daydreaming.

After our patient leaves, I'm typing my notes when it hits me again, this time it's the real deal. I double over on my chair, unable to breathe. A deep visceral pain that overwhelms my senses and paralyses my whole body. Maybe I don't have the highest pain threshold, I've never experienced childbirth as a means for comparison, but to this day, this is the worst pain I have suffered. It felt like someone using eagle-beak forceps to remove my intestines via my mouth. This time it didn't go unnoticed. 'You're not alright, are you?' Lorraine's voice still sounded muffled through my ringing ears. I of course replied, 'yeah, I'll be fine'.

I wasn't alright. I'd pushed myself too hard, too soon.

I couldn't suppress my eagerness and ego to slow down and grow steadily. I wanted to be the best, the best dentist, for myself and my patients. I believed I could be the best within a few short years by pushing myself harder and harder, at the expense of everything else, including my health.

The crippling cramps repeated hourly for several weeks. Having tried and failed to ignore it, not telling anyone and trying not to make a fuss, I went to the doctor. The antispasmodics didn't help. A colonoscopy didn't find anything either. At least it's not serious I thought, just the incapacitating pain then. It felt as though this could be me now, for the long term, I may just have to learn to deal with it.

I realised that the cause which is so obvious now, was stress. I had wanted to be a dentist since the age of 15 and put all my energy into getting here, to find that maybe I couldn't handle the stress, maybe it wasn't worth the mental anguish and physical ramifications. Maybe I needed to get out of dentistry altogether, cut my losses and do something I really loved. Something that wasn't going to send me to an early grave. I still felt I was good at what I was doing and I still wanted to be the best, but I was doing something wrong, I just couldn't work out what it was.

Life carried on in much the same way until Christmas, about 2 am on the 24th of December, following the staff Christmas do to be more precise. A friend had dropped me off outside my flat and I simply had to overcome my intoxication for a few moments to traverse the icy slope to the front door of the apartment block and into bed. I'm not sure whether the ice on the floor or the ice in my drink was more to blame, but I do remember the moment I slipped and the full weight of my body went through my left elbow to the tarmac below. The stress breaker was my humerus, which now had an oblique displaced fracture.

Sat sobering in the hospital, I tried to come to terms with the sheer idiocy of what I'd done and the pain I was probably going to be in tomorrow. My ego was bruised, my arm broken and my new career unburgeoned. In one moment I'd gone from feeling like a flourishing dentist to being unable to load my toothbrush.

I was faced with a choice between spending three months unable to work with my arm in a sling or having surgery with a 15% risk of damaging my radial nerve, potentially ending my career before it had even really begun. To complicate the decision, I was warned that if I missed a quarter of my foundation year, there was a good chance I'd have to start my post-graduate training all over again. It's telling of where my true passion lay, that in that moment I was most concerned that if the surgery went wrong, I wouldn't be able to play piano. The quick fix is rarely the best solution and so I braced myself for the longer road ahead.

With my arm in a sling and time on my hands, I began to reflect on the path I was on and what I truly wanted to do with my career. I spent time travelling around, shadowing as many different dentists in as many different locations as possible. Everything from high-end implant and cosmetic dentistry, oral surgery, orthodontics, through general dentistry and into the community, including some intriguing days shadowing dentists helping those kept at Her Majesty's pleasure.

The most important thing I discovered during this time was that my stomach cramps had disappeared. My literal break from dentisting had revealed that my career was breaking me and it only took my complete incapacitation to realise this. I had the opportunity to stop, reflect, and reevaluate what matters most to me and where I was going. Breaking my arm was the best thing that happened to me, I found so many opportunities during this time, I gained exposure to sides of dentistry I would have never thought about and I wouldn't be who I am today if it hadn't happened.

The time I'd been given allowed me a period of introspection, a chance to grow and develop in ways that I would never have managed if I'd still been blitzing through a list of NHS patients. I was lucky to be working at Glencairn Dental Practice, where the principal dentists were placing a lot of dental implants and this is where my fascination with implantology was born. I was lucky to have close friends and family who supported me and a small but valuable network of dentists to turn to for guidance. Fortune seems to have followed me a lot through my career so far, though of course, breaking my arm didn't feel like good luck at the time. The ensuing years have been coloured by thousands more incidents and mistakes that often feel traumatic, but have shaped who I am today.

In this book, I hope to give you the tools you need to find your passion and build a fulfilling career in dentistry. Austin Kleon told us that 'all advice is autobiographical' and much of what you will read is what I wish I'd understood a long time ago. I love being a dentist, but I haven't always felt this way. There have been sleepless nights and painful days. I left dental school with a desire to care for patients, only to become rapidly overwhelmed by the pressure I put on myself to be perfect, the fear of regulation and litigation, and the chasm between the work I was doing and what I saw on social media. I questioned how much longer I'd be able to carry on being a dentist and the answer certainly wasn't forty more years.

I've delved deeply into my mental wellbeing, enduring periods of lows that some people may identify with, but I hope that even those who've never felt this way, will gain something from sharing my experiences. There is more to fixing teeth than filling holes, just as there's more to life than dentistry. This book is written with the belief that we all have the tools to thrive in our careers and we can do so in a way that maintains a balance in our lives for what matters most.

Nobody is born with a raging desire to fix teeth and you don't need to break your arm to discover your passion. You do need to be ready to put in the work, reflect on your core values and learn from your mistakes. I hope this book can fan the flames of your passion whether you are just starting out, if you've fallen out of love with dentistry, or if you already have a passion that you want to burn as brightly as possible. My passion is what drives me not to be the best anymore, but to be my best, for my patients, my family, and myself.

It's been over twelve years since a muggy day in Liverpool which marked my graduation from dental school, with a modest amount of knowledge about holes in teeth and a little experience of patching them up again. In those years, I've learned quite a bit more about teeth and a lot more about life. I've found my passion in dentistry and I'm not the only one. Thousands of people in dentistry love what they do and with this book, I want to share with you the secrets to finding a passion so you too can be In The Loupe.

# 1

# There Must Be More to Life Than This

Freddie Mercury

## *How to find your purpose*

"I slept and dreamt that life was joy. I awoke and saw that life was service. I acted and behold, service was joy."
**Rabindranath Tagore**

*When I came to see Karl, I had lost all confidence in my smile. I'd developed habits to hide my teeth and I never showed my teeth when I smiled for photos. When I was five, I was diagnosed with amelogenesis imperfecta and by the time I was ten, I had my first set of NHS veneers. At the time the aesthetics meant nothing to me, but by the time I reached my early twenties, my teeth were uneven, different sizes and slanted down to one side when I smiled. I decided life was too short to smile with my hand over my mouth, that's when I came to see Karl. I explained my insecurities and he came up with a plan to give me my smile back. When the final veneers were fitted I could have cried with happiness. After so many years of being so self-conscious about my teeth, I finally found and fell in love with my smile again.*

I have always enjoyed helping people, like many dentists, it's one of the reasons I chose to study dentistry. As a newly qualified dentist, I enjoyed the satisfaction of getting people out of pain and helping them to have healthy teeth, but treating Nic was a turning point in my career. This was more than just a patient telling me that they used to be scared but now they're not, I realised that I'd made a real difference in her life. When Nic comes back to see me, smiling and full of confidence, she's a different person and this fills me with an enormous sense of pride. For the first time, I felt that I hadn't just fixed someone's teeth I'd helped them as a person.

The skills I needed to undertake Nic's treatment took several years for me to develop and required a highly skilled team of people around me to deliver it over the course of a year. It wasn't the complexity of the treatment that mattered though, the real significance of Nic's treatment was the time I'd spent getting to know Nic, understanding who she was and how I could help her. Most patients don't need a full rehabilitation, but every patient is a human who we have the opportunity to help, not merely by checking for holes and filling them, but by forming a genuine connection with the person the mouth is attached to.

Seeing the difference I'd made to Nic was when I first felt I had a real purpose in what I was doing. It's this purpose that is fundamental to everything I do now, which direction I want my career to take, how I'm going to get there, and why I'm doing it. My purpose is what pulls me through the difficult times and drives me forward in the good. When I first qualified I believed that having the motivation to want to do my best for my patients and a will to better myself was all I needed to sustain my growth. However, I now see the real power that comes from having a clearly defined purpose. It was helping Nic that crystallised this, but if I had stopped and taken the time to reflect on what really matters to me, I could have found my purpose much earlier in my career.

While I have always been keen to improve my skills, attending courses and joining societies, I have wasted a great deal of money and lost many hours on things that have been of no use to me. It's not that they were bad courses or that I didn't meet some great people, just that they didn't have any real benefit for me or my career. Sometimes I learned things that I never used and so forgot, other times it was the right course, just done at the wrong time. I'd book onto these courses in a blaze of excitement thinking the more I do, the better I'll get, with no regard for whether they'd actually help me in the right way. I did this because I didn't understand why I was doing anything, other than wanting to get better.

The Olympic gold medal winning rower Ben Hunt-Davis didn't have this problem. He and his team knew the only thing that mattered in the run-up to the Sydney Olympics in 2000 was doing everything in their power to win a gold medal. Each member of the Men's Eight rowing team asked themselves, before every single thing they did, at home, in the gym, or on the lake, 'will it make the boat go faster?' In the six months leading up to that race, that was the only thing that mattered to them. If they could not answer 'yes' to that question, then they didn't do it.

Ben and his team existed on the extreme end of living with purpose, where every action they took was focused on one clearly defined goal which was the only thing that mattered to them at that time, at the cost of everything else in their lives. We're not in a sprint for a gold medal, but it's the same understanding of a purpose that will empower us to maximise our potential. To sustain a passion in the long term, we need to find fulfilment in our careers. Understanding our purpose will help us develop in the right direction, avoid wasting time on endeavours that don't actually help us, and lift us when we find obstacles on our path.

## Losing my Motivation

I have always considered myself to be a driven person, someone who needs no external pressures to keep pushing forward, but this proved untrue as I catastrophically failed my exams in my second year of dental school. The reason was obvious, I'd done no work all year. I had lost the drive that I had taken for granted. It's not that I didn't want to do well, I had just taken my foot off the pedal, coasting along and for some reason, I was surprised when I came to a halt.

Growing up, I had always worked hard in school, I wanted to do well for myself but like most kids, I wanted to make my parents proud. I loved seeing the pride in my mum's eyes when she told her friends that her son was going to be a dentist. When I got to university, living in halls, that motivator suddenly disappeared. I had thrived on being one of the brightest kids in the class but now I was just one of many, in fact, I felt like I was surrounded by students who were much smarter than me. I had worked harder in school to stay ahead of the rest but now, in the middle to lower order, I didn't see the point in doing anything more than was necessary to get by. Besides this, spending time with friends and drinking was more enjoyable than studying.

I passed my first year on the back of the work I did for my A levels, which encouraged me to do even less work in second year. My work ethic had evaporated and the exams had got harder, I only realised this as I walked out of the end-of-year exam and for the first time in my life, I knew I'd failed. A comprehension of my transgressions hit me like a sledgehammer. My failure was humiliating, particularly as it was entirely my own fault, but worse than the embarrassment, I felt lost. I had lost sight of why I was studying to be a dentist and who I was doing it for. That summer, before the cramming for the resits could begin, I had to reflect on what I was doing with my life and why I was doing it. I couldn't just coast along anymore.

This all happened two years before Simon Sinek would publish Start With Why and it would be a long time before I treated Nic and discovered what dentistry was really about for me. I realised at that time that I had to do this for me and nobody else. Parental pride certainly wasn't going to sustain a career. Dentistry could offer me a lifestyle that I wanted, I knew I had the academic ability and the manual dexterity to do it and most importantly, I would get to help people every day. It felt selfish to focus on myself and what I could get out of it, but I knew it was right for me at the time and I was the only person who could make it happen. It's only through mastering ourselves that we can truly be at our best to help others.

What I unearthed was renewed a desire to push myself, not to be better than anyone else, just to be the best I could be. I attacked my studies with renewed vigour, finding that the motivation that came from within was far stronger than anything I'd felt before. I still managed to take time out to enjoy myself, going to Leeds Festival a couple of weeks before the resits, but I went knowing that I'd bust a gut all summer to get back on track. Invigorated by this realisation, I felt empowered and ready to take on the world again.

Doing things for personal gain, however, was not likely to sustain me for a lifetime. I knew that my ultimate aim was to help people and I knew that I wanted to work towards something greater than myself. Viktor Frankl, the psychiatrist and Holocaust survivor, found that the people who survived the longest through the atrocities of the concentration camps were those, including himself, who had a self-transcending purpose. A purpose that goes beyond ourselves and is driven by what we can give to the world leads to sustainably higher levels of motivation.

When John F Kennedy visited the NASA Space Centre in 1962, he interrupted his tour to speak to a janitor. 'Hi, I'm Jack Kennedy' he said, 'what are you doing?' 'I'm helping to put a man on the moon, Mr President' came the janitor's reply. This janitor's appreciation that he was part of something much bigger than himself, much more than sweeping the floor, gave him a sense of fulfilment and passion about what he was doing. These disparate tales, one of a holocaust survivor, and another of an American cleaner couldn't be more divergent in context, and yet they are characterised by the same understanding that they are a part of something bigger than them as individuals.

I know that I'm not going to single-handedly change the world, but by helping each of my patients, by giving them confidence in their teeth and their smile, I can make the world a slightly better place. I know that each of those patients will be able to go and live their best lives and I've been able to play my small part in the much bigger picture.

"He who has a why to live for can bear almost any how."
**Friedrich Nietzsche**

We all have our own purpose, it may be similar to others, but what motivates each of us will be slightly different, based on our unique life experiences. As time passes, our experiences and our priorities in life change, and our purpose will change too. Taking the time for introspection, to find our purpose will lay the foundations from which we can grow. Every day that I work on clinic, every training opportunity I seek, and every holiday I take, is done with an appreciation of my purpose.

Your purpose will not dictate your life plan, but it will inform what you do from this day forward. It will draw on your deepest values and these will be unique to you. It will guide you towards the right path when there's a fork in the road. It will be your mantra that will give you strength in difficult times and it will become the seed from which your passion will grow.

## How I Found My Purpose

Anyone can tell you what they do, some can tell you how they do it, but most people can't tell you why they do it. Our purpose is the why, and finding it takes time and reflection. It's not something that trips off the tongue after thirty seconds of musing and it's about more than the distilled words that may form your final mantra. Finding our purpose is about a process of introspection, it's about honestly reflecting on who we are, what our values and motivations are and what matters to us above all else. For the purposes of this exercise, I'm going to use the role of the dentist as the subject, but you can replace this with any role inside or outside of healthcare.

I want you to start by taking a minute to think back to just before you started university, to a time when you told people you were going to study dentistry and people would ask you why, usually accompanied by the lines 'I could never do that', 'why would you want to look in people's mouths all day' and the immortal 'good money though, eh' [nudge nudge wink wink]. You probably had a stock answer ready each time and it probably lost all meaning once you'd repeated it for the hundredth time. That stock answer came from somewhere though. Take a moment to reflect on these questions:

Why did you want to study dentistry?
What values do you hold inside that made you give these reasons for getting into dentistry?

These answers will start to help you to realise your core values and what being a dentist means to you, even if your perceptions about what dentistry is have changed from what you thought it would be. Your reasons for choosing dentistry and your underlying values will be different to mine because your experiences are different to mine. We live our lives according to the conscious and subconscious stories we tell ourselves about who we are. We form these stories through our lived experiences and by reflecting on the most significant ones, we can uncover a deeper understanding of what motivates us.

Once you've got a few answers to these warm-up questions, it's time to dig a little deeper. Forgetting about your occupation now, I want you to think about and write down as many stories as possible that tell me about who you are. These stories can be about anything from any time, from early childhood to the present day. They may be vivid memories or experiences in which you can't remember all the details but you can remember the way you felt. Your stories don't always need to be positive and sometimes they're even painful to think about, what matters is taking the time to acknowledge them and that they're a part of who you are today. They may take you weeks to come up with and it will help to note down as many as you can. Here are a few examples of my own.

*I have always enjoyed helping people. At the tender age of four and a half, I was the eldest of four children. I always felt it was my responsibility to help look after my younger siblings and I thrived believing that I was doing my part to help them and support my parents.*

*My Grandad told me of how his family travelled back and forth between the UK and the US during the Great Depression, as the work dried up and his father was struggling to put food on the table. I remember having a fear of that vulnerability, not knowing where the money for the next meal might come from. I'm generally risk-averse and I realised that I wanted to make a living in a more stable way that would allow me to provide for my family.*

*I remember marvelling at how hard my dad worked, leaving before I got up for breakfast every morning and getting home after tea, just to provide for his family. I also remember feeling that I just wanted to spend more time with him. I knew that I would want to be as present as possible for my kids and that family would always be at the heart of my life.*

These little parcels of emotion are a sample of the many that I felt were relevant to me, there were many more, some deeply personal, others seemingly trivial, but they all stick in my memory and on some level, influence who I am today. I found it helpful to share my stories with my wife, Marisa, which as well as helping me understand what was important in them, gave us a wonderful opportunity to connect. Marisa also suggested other stories I'd told her that I'd not mentioned and helped me reflect on their significance to me.

Once you have collected as many stories as you can, it's time to start thinking more deeply about them. Read back through your stories and try to find the common themes, notice how you feel when you recount them and identify what values each story represents. My stories are experiences that have stuck with me over the years because they define who I am, they are meaningful to me and they shape my values to this day. Try to identify one or two core values in each of your stories and notice which values appear most frequently. In my stories, I found values of honesty, family, security and responsibility, amongst others. If you need help identifying what constitutes a value, search for Brené Brown's Dare to Lead List of Values.

Another way to find which values are important to you is to picture yourself at your own funeral, your family are there, as are your friends and your colleagues. What are they saying about you? What do you want them to say? These two questions often have very different answers.

Our values aren't necessarily set in stone, they are simply a product of our life experiences. We do not emerge from the womb with rigidly fixed values. This means that as our life changes and we have new experiences, our values can change. We also have the power to change the values we don't like. If by undertaking this process of reflection you uncover some values that conflict with who you want to be, you have the power to change them. We create new stories about ourselves every day. If there are values that you would like to have, ask yourself 'how would someone who embodies these values act?' You are not tied into a contract with your values, you get to dictate the terms and become the person you want to be.

Once you've created your list of core values, whittle the list down to the five that feel most important to you, these are probably the values that came up most in your stories. You're going to use these values now to write your purpose. Express it however feels right to you, but often this will take the form of 'To..... so that.....'

My purpose, which evolved over several weeks and many hours of reflection is:

**"To help people by restoring confidence in their smile in a friendly and professional manner and to inspire others to do the same, so that the people I help can positively influence those around them."**

My values have informed this mantra, though not all of them will be immediately apparent to anyone else reading it. I'm reminded of my core values when I read it and it serves to keep me focused on the things that matter most to me. My purpose is about me, but it's also about what I can do for the people I come into contact with. It's not a rigidly defined goal, but an infinite purpose that represents what matters most at this point in time.

Finding your purpose will take time and deep thought. It won't be the same as mine, though there are likely to be similarities for most people working in healthcare. Nothing is ever perfect right away and your purpose can, and will, evolve. It's the process of discovering our purpose that is more important than the final words on the page.

Write your purpose down and put it somewhere that you will see it every day. Remind yourself of it every morning and come back to it when you're feeling depleted. Some cyclists harness the power of their purpose by writing it on their handlebars. When they feel their tank is empty, their head drops and they look down, their purpose is written in plain sight to remind them why they're doing this, giving them the strength to push on. You can keep it on your phone, print it on your water bottle, the bottom of your mug, or write it in glow-in-the-dark ink on the wall in the dark cupboard that you lock yourself in when the world outside gets a bit too much.

By understanding and articulating my purpose, I can use it to decide how I'm going to go about being a dentist. What do I need to do to be able to fulfil my purpose? Which courses do I need to go on? Which skills do I want to develop? When I'm at my best, how do I act and what do I do? How can I create an environment to help me thrive? Not only does my purpose help me to answer these questions, but by understanding my purpose, I can be open with my patients about what motivates me and this has had a profound impact too.

# Purpose in Practice

It was after articulating my purpose that I accidentally brought David, a work-hardened middle-aged bloke, to tears. I was mentoring a student on the MSc in Dental Implantology programme at ICE in Salford. He had completed his assessment and identified that some complex restorative work, beyond his current skillset, would be required before David could have dental implants. David had come to the hospital for a cheaper dental implant and now the treatment going to take a lot longer and cost a lot more than he'd hoped. He was understandably upset and frustrated, he didn't think he could afford the treatment that was necessary to get him functioning and smiling again. The student brought me, as the mentor on clinic, to talk to David and give my opinion.

I listened to David as he explained to me what he wanted from his treatment, he just wanted to be able to smile again without the big gaps. He had lost all confidence, not only in his teeth but in himself, and now the ideal affordable solution had been taken away from him. He didn't ask for dental implants. He didn't ask for new crowns. He just wanted to be able to smile again.

I explained to him that what matters most to me, is giving my patients a smile they could be proud of, not just by plugging the holes with a few screws, but by considering what is going to allow them to smile with confidence for many years to come. I explained to him what would be involved in doing this for him, how it would take around a year and a rough estimate of the costs, which were into five figures. I explained that the moment that means the most to me is at the end of treatment when my patient gets to look in the mirror and see their new teeth for the first time. How they often give their first real smile for many years, a smile that gives them back their confidence and their life.

As I explained this to a guy that had hardly let his face slip all appointment, I saw his eyes start to fill up, which of course nearly always gets me going. David could see that I'd truly listened and understood what truly mattered to him. This happy, friendly, dad had spent so long hiding his teeth that he'd almost forgotten how to smile. Just the thought of being able to get back to that, to be able to laugh and play with his kids without inhibition meant everything.

By taking the time to understand my patient and not just focusing on his teeth, by knowing my purpose and being able to talk openly about it, I had the opportunity to help this wonderful man and give him a new lease of life. Not every patient requires a call to arms like David, and we must be careful not to overpromise or attempt to provide work beyond our competency under the guise of trying to help. But if we've listened empathically and understood what matters to our patients, we'll be able to connect deeply with them and offer them the kind of care that can change their lives and in turn provide us with the foundations of a fulfilling career.

# Coda

| Three steps to mastery |
| --- |
| 1. Allocate time to stop and reflect on the stories that have shaped who you are. |
| 2. Uncover the values in these stories by reflecting and sharing them. |
| 3. Use your core values to formulate your purpose and remind yourself of it every day. |

Passion begins with purpose. If we don't understand why we're doing something, we will never have the drive to keep moving forward. Understanding your purpose will lay the foundations for everything that follows in this book. I spent a lot of time in my early years bouncing around different areas of dentistry, some of this was exploration, but much was simply because I hadn't taken the time to reflect on what really mattered to me. By finding my purpose I've been able to work with much greater focus and I've found my work to be more fulfilling. I use my purpose as a grounding for my decision making and in doing so, I am making decisions that keep me rooted to my core values. We each have our own unique purpose and it's only through dedicated introspection that we can begin to understand it.

The first draft of your purpose will usually be in the form of 'To..... so that.....' I use the word draft very deliberately, this is not final, it does not have to be perfect and you will want to review your purpose throughout your life as you have new experiences that change your values. It's the process of inquisition that matters more than the final words on the page.

I remind myself of my purpose every day. It reinforces the work I do and gives me strength on difficult days. My purpose also gives my life direction, helping me to decide the best use of my time so I'm in control of where I'm going.

# 2

# Runnin' Down a Dream

## Tom Petty and the Heartbreakers

### *How to give your life direction*

"You can hit 10,000 golf balls and never get any better if
you don't know where they're going."
**Matthew Syed**

What does a great dentist look like? Are you already a
great dentist? Maybe you're going to be a great dentist,
you know you want to get there but also, you're aware you
don't have the skills and experience yet. This position of
ambition and uncertainty is a beautiful place to be, and I
hope it's a place you never leave. It's from this place that
you will keep driving to be better. I think I'm quite a good
dentist, I certainly strive to be. I've grown a lot in my
career and yet I know there is still so much more to learn.

The great dentists are not the ones who perform the grandest, most elaborate treatment plans, but the ones who show up every day and consistently provide excellent care for their patients. If we want to become great dentists, in every interaction with a patient or colleague, every stage of a treatment plan, and every step of the patient journey, we need to do the small things well.

It's easy to get caught up in our own little world, letting tiredness, stress or fatigue get the better of us, and this can impact our decision-making and our performance. If we want to maintain a high level of performance even when we're not at our best, it can help to ask ourselves what the great dentist we envisage in our head would do in this situation. What we may feel like doing at 5 pm on a Friday is not always the same as what we'd expect a great dentist to do and viewing the situation from an external perspective can aid us in making the right decision to provide the best possible care for our patients.

We can fall into the trap of thinking we need to gather all the knowledge and all the skills before magically becoming the perfect dentist but it's the small things we do today that set us on the right path for tomorrow. We have all had times when we've placed a filling and it's broken the same day because we had failed to check the occlusion properly. It's a small but vitally important step that we can put right immediately and when it happens again in the future, which of course, it will at some point, we can reflect with pride on how infrequently it happens now, when perhaps it used to be a regular occurrence.

I can see now that the time I used to spend fire-fighting fractured cusps was because I hadn't assessed and protected the vulnerable teeth appropriately. Identifying my earlier failings gives me confidence that I'm moving in the right direction. The same is true looking forwards, there are probably things that I do now that one day I will look back on and think I should have done better and that's ok too. We are better for knowing that we can do better. We will never be perfect, even those dentists who we believe are at the top of their game will know they can keep improving.

There will be no single moment in our career when we will be able to say we have mastered every aspect of it. There may be achievements and accolades along the way, but we are on a perpetual journey and at no point will anyone be declared the winner of dentistry. The moment we retire will not be the moment of our greatest achievement and so we can't compare our career to climbing a mountain or running a marathon where there is a clear finish line.

Our career is what has come to be known as an infinite game. The purpose of an infinite game is to keep playing, to keep enjoying it and to keep doing a little bit better as you go. Our purpose should also be infinite, there should be no definitive endpoint. As we keep improving, the world around us keeps changing and we can make further improvements still. There is no point in setting a fixed destination for our career because the path we're walking down is constantly changing just as we're changing as we take it.

"You don't have to see the whole staircase, just take the first step."
**Martin Luther King Jr**

If we were to draw a map of our life's journey today, we would have to choose a destination based on our current knowledge. We would follow a single path, without deviation, to a fixed place. This destination accounts for none of the obstacles we will encounter and none of the better paths that we may find. It doesn't account for the moment we discover that the destination we are heading towards isn't all it's cracked up to be. It doesn't account for the moment when we realise we've been holding the map upside down and what we thought the world looked like is all backwards and doesn't make sense any more. The map of our lives isn't even static, it changes constantly, and so our destination is always moving.

My childhood dentist didn't always wear gloves when he checked my teeth, a pile of used instruments would sit in the corner of the worktop somewhere near the autoclave, next to a half-eaten apple and three tankards of tea, empty but for the indelible brown scars at the base. This antediluvian dentistry was less than thirty years ago and the *absurd* changes such as clean gloves for every patient were met with resistance by some across the dental team at the time.

Further improvements during our careers are inevitable, some of which may seem radical and will be met with the same resistance. There's every chance that in thirty years we'll be reflecting on something with the same incredulity as we view not wearing gloves now. Just because this is the way things are done now, does not mean it's right and it certainly doesn't mean this is how things are going to be done in the future.

We need to create a system that allows for the changing world around us rather than overlooking it. In a world that is constantly improving, if we're not changing for the better, we're getting worse. It's time to get rid of the old model of a career map and the fixed destination fallacy. Instead let's use our purpose, formed from our core values, as our compass to guide us on a changing landscape. Let's move on from the myopic drive to get closer to the prize at the end of the rope and focus on taking one step at a time in the right direction.

# Direction

By using our purpose as our compass, we can be confident we're heading towards our true north and we then have the freedom to enjoy the journey, precisely because we're not fixated on the destination. We can start to make a difference today, making the world around us a little bit better for the people within it. In dentistry, we have the opportunity to make a positive impact on dozens of lives every day, with our patients, our team, our family and our friends. Patients come to us for help and we get to use our unique set of skills to make their lives better, it's by focusing on our strengths that we can start to see where we may be able to have the biggest impact and use our skills in the best way.

We all have strengths and weaknesses. When we want to start improving ourselves, we often seek to plug the holes by identifying our weaknesses, yet nobody has ever done well in life by being fairly good at everything. We succeed, not because we don't have any weaknesses, but because we play to our strengths. We need to have an awareness of both to thrive and taking the time to reflect on these strengths and weaknesses will be key in helping us in setting our life's direction.

You can start setting your direction by answering the following questions:

1.  If I keep doing what I'm doing, what will my life look like in 5, 10 or 20 years?
2.  What do I currently do that I'm not very good at?
3.  What do I currently do that I hate?
4.  What am I better at than most other people in my position?
5.  What do I love doing?
6.  What do I do that when doing it, I feel completely focused and like I'm doing my best work?

When you answer these questions, keep in mind that soft skills like communication, creativity and adaptability are as important, if not more important than technical skills and knowledge in dentistry. Don't stop at a list of answers, reflect and expand upon them. Explain why you've given each answer and delve into the specifics of what it is that you love or hate.

How do these answers fit in with your purpose? With each answer, you will gain some clarity and the more colour you can add to your answer, the stronger your understanding will be. Here are a couple of examples of my own from 2014:

*I'm working five days a week, four and a half are entirely NHS, mostly check-ups, with half a day of implants. I'm also spending extra time outside of work studying for my master's and my wife is pregnant with our first child. I often feel very stressed and I'm having to do a lot of my treatment plans on top of my clinical hours. If I carry on like this, in the next 10 years I'm going to have very little time with my family and I will probably burn out completely.*

*I hate how little time I get with most of my patients. I love building great relationships with them as I do with my implant patients, I have the time to get to know them and I feel like I can really help them. I can work quickly but I don't think the quality of my work is as good as it could be when I do so. I want to do work that makes a bigger difference to people and I want to have more time to spend with my family.*

Using these reflections I was able to see that my future lay away from a fast-paced environment and that working five clinical days a week was too much for me. Understanding this, I could reset my compass, directing my career towards one that would play to my strengths and allow me to enjoy the most important parts of my life. What shortly followed was our relocation across the

Pennines, leaving my old jobs on the Wirral and landing my first job in private practice in Yorkshire. A few years later, I wrote these:

*I've enjoyed the opportunities to teach on the implant nurses' course. I was really nervous before doing it but felt ok once I got going. The feedback from the days I've done has been really good, though I know I can get better with more practice.*

*I enjoy placing dental implants and I'd like to do more but I also enjoy seeing my regular patients coming back to me and the long-term relationships I have with them.*

*I love seeing the difference that treatments like dental implants can make for my patients and I want to do more work that has a bigger difference for them. I find formulating longer treatment plans difficult but I can do it well when I've got the time to do it properly.*

These reflections in 2018 highlighted that I wanted to do more comprehensive dentistry, though not necessarily fixated on surgical implant treatment. I reset my compass and began looking for courses and mentors that would help me grow in this new direction.

By first finding our purpose, then reflecting on our current situation, we can begin to set out in the right direction. Taking small purposeful steps will help us in the long term to grow and enjoy our journey. One of the secrets to finding a passion in dentistry, therefore, is not to focus on finding a passion but to work on the steps that can help us build a fulfilling career for ourselves. Passion, just like other labels such as happiness or success are not destinations on a map, they're the outcomes of the things we choose to do, day in and day out.

## Outcomes

Outcomes are the successes or failures that happen to us. They are beyond our control because they are affected by an infinite number of external factors. We can delight a patient with a terrible denture if the patient has low expectations, but this doesn't mean we're good at making dentures. Similarly, we can make a brilliant denture that a patient hates and this doesn't mean we're useless. Rather than focusing on the outcome of the treatment, we can work on the process. A terrible denture that a patient is happy with means little if we fail to improve our process. If we can focus on our processes and take steps to make small improvements every time we do something, the outcomes will take care of themselves.

Seth Godin, American business legend and author of many thought-provoking books, taught me how to juggle. He taught me that catching is not the problem. Focusing on catching, the outcome, is what makes us start to lunge for the ball and the moment we do this, it's game over. The real issue is throwing. If we can learn how to throw the ball in the right direction, with the right weight, then the catching will take care of itself. So, we learn to throw a ball perfectly first, we throw the ball and let it fall to the ground. We learn to accept the uncomfortable truth that it's ok to drop the ball. When we can throw one ball consistently in the right place, we throw two balls, again letting them both fall to the ground.

By focusing on the process of throwing and not worrying about the outcome, catching, we learn to get the most important part right first. Once we're throwing the balls in the right place, catching them is a lot easier. Finally, when we're ready, we can add a third ball. Like learning any new skill, we won't be perfect straight away, but developing the process instead of focusing on the outcome works a lot better than any other system.

By focusing on the process, we can start to make meaningful, long-lasting changes to our lives. In my early years, I believed that becoming a great dentist would require epochs of continuing professional development (CPD) to improve my technical skills. I would take the most spectacular courses but they were often beyond my clinical ability. I was still figuring out how to predictably place fillings that didn't create food traps and I was on a course about using synthetic bone augmentation materials to gain vertical bone height for dental implants. While what I saw was inspiring, the majority of it went straight over my head and has been of no use to me since.

It would have been more useful in my formative years to focus on developing my clinical skills by deliberate practice appropriate to the level of knowledge I'd left university with, in addition to working on my communication skills, which are essential if we want to truly help our patients. Alongside this, I could have spent time on personal development and growing as a person to allow me to fulfil my potential outside of clinic.

Life is about more than teeth and by broadening our horizons beyond our dental surroundings we will become better dentists. Nobody wants to go for a drink with the person who is so immersed in their daily grind that they have nothing else to talk about. It makes building rapport with anyone impossible, whether it's colleagues, patients or friends.

Though I didn't realise it at the time, the skills I needed to become better at clinical dentistry are the same skills I developed when learning to play piano, things like focus, listening, persistence, manual dexterity and rest. As a timid child, often bullied and outcast, it was playing the piano and performing that gave me strength and confidence. Now as an educator, I can translate this confidence to stand up in front of a room full of people to teach and inspire. It doesn't happen overnight but by keeping varied interests in life we will develop skills that help us grow in ways we cannot always see in the moment.

## Reflection

Reflection has already made up a large part of how we're going to set our direction, by unearthing our values and helping us to articulate our purpose. We're going to use reflection now to help with more specific events and to refine our processes. Self-awareness is what separates us from other animals but it's a gift that we often choose not to use. By honestly appraising ourselves we can supercharge our learning and avoid repeating our mistakes. Reflection is about dedicating a small amount of time regularly, to look at ourselves so we can improve, for our own fulfilment and in turn, so we can better help the people around us.

"The unexamined life is not worth living."
**Socrates**

Reflection allows us to discover our hidden strengths and weaknesses. We can identify what has worked well and where there are still areas for improvement. Reflection after a course also provides a moment of quiet contemplation to draw out the most valuable lessons so we can implement them in practice. By revisiting my course notes a day or two after, I can identify the most salient points and put them into action.

I reflect on treatments that have gone particularly well and certainly on those that haven't turned out the way I'd hoped, why they happened and how I'm going to improve my process going forwards. I reflect and learn from times when I've confused a patient by giving too many options or said something with good intentions that's had the wrong effect. Reflections can also be of non-clinical events, interactions with team members, personal performance, stress or time management and professionalism.

A template for your own reflections can be downloaded from WalkerFinch.com/resources.

The six prompts I use for reflection are based on the Gibbs Reflective Cycle. These are:

1. Description. What happened?
2. Feelings. How did you feel before, during and after the event?
3. Evaluation. What went well? What didn't?
4. Analysis. Why did this happen?
5. Conclusion. What did you learn?
6. Action plan. What are you going to do differently from now on?

There is no point in education or practice without reflection. If we don't take the time to critically reflect on our work and our life, we will never improve. It's this process of reflection that then feeds back into our direction. Once we've reflected, we can amend our direction to further improve, whether it's by identifying an area that we want to move away from, or an area we'd like to seek further improvement in. This reflection and direction cycle is ongoing throughout our careers, the journey of self-improvement is never completed.

# Coda

| Three steps to mastery |
| --- |
| 1. Use the questions on page 32 along with your purpose to help set you on the right path towards your own true north. |
| 2. When your direction is set, focus on improving your processes, don't become fixated on your outcomes. |
| 3. Allocate time to regularly reflect on specific events to further refine your processes. |

Our purpose is our compass, guiding us in the right direction on a changing landscape, freeing us from the fixed mindset of a rigidly set destination. In this way, we are free from the shackles of uncontrollable outcomes, to improve our process and enjoy the journey. It's important to start by improving our self-awareness, taking the time to reflect on where we are now, our strengths and weaknesses, so we can correctly calibrate our compass. By focusing on the process, the small steps we take on our journey, we can continually improve and in doing so the outcome, our destination, will take care of itself.

Actively engage with the process of reflection by dedicating a small amount of time regularly to it. Use this reflection along with your purpose to set your direction without fixating on a specific outcome. Once you're facing in the right direction, you're ready to take the first step in improving your process.

# 3
# Little by Little
## Oasis

### *How to harness the power of habits*

"You can't connect the dots looking forward. You can only connect them looking backwards. You have to trust that the dots will somehow connect in your future."
**Steve Jobs**

We are hard-wired to love immediate gratification, that little flutter of excitement that we get with likes on social media, eating chocolate or achieving our short-term goals. That flutter is dopamine, the feel-good hormone that's released when we consume high-energy food or survive a dangerous situation. Homo sapiens needed this reward system to survive 30,000 years ago, it's what told us what was good to eat and what would keep us alive.

The problem is that our hormones haven't evolved at the same rate as the world around us and so our bodies can't tell the difference between nutritious fruit and chocolate or, escaping a lion and receiving likes for an Instagram post. It's no surprise then that we get hooked on junk food and doom scrolling, we have evolved to crave the sensation dopamine gives us but it does little for us in the long term in our modern lives. Activities that provide an immediate pay-off in the form of dopamine rarely provide positive long-lasting benefits. Real growth comes from making small improvements every day and often these don't come with instant gratification. Real growth happens when we forgo the quick pay-off and focus on maximising our effectiveness day upon day. In this way, we incrementally grow a little stronger and it's only in retrospect that we may start to see a significant difference and how it all fits together.

## Goals

If we've established a clear direction and a purpose, we do not also need to set ourselves goals. Goals are modern hacks that encourage us to create arbitrary targets to give ourselves that dopamine hit when we achieve them. Goals can focus our mind on a singular task but they lack any emphasis on quality and in narrowing our focus, they distract us from everything else that's going on, sequestering us from other opportunities. The process of setting ourselves goals can encourage reflection and planning but we can dedicate time for introspection to find our purpose and regularly review our direction without them.

I spent years setting myself goals in the pursuit of professional development, 'I want to place 50 implants next year' was a persistent favourite. It feels good when we achieve a goal of course, but that little spike of dopamine doesn't last long and then what? We can either bask in our own radiant glory or set another goal and start again. In the push to hit our target, we may have been so focused on reaching the destination that we didn't learn from the steps we took along the way. By focusing solely on the outcome, we neglect the process. I could have achieved my target of placing 50 implants a year much quicker if I'd taken a bit less time on each case, if I'd have compromised my values and advised an implant when a bonded bridge was more suitable, if I'd stayed on clinic instead of going on more courses, or if I'd worked six days a week, but at what cost?

Goals are the waypoints on a map with a specific destination in mind but as we travel through life, the map changes. When the rules of the game change, the biggest losers are the people who are still trying to play by the old rules. When online movie streaming came to the fore, Blockbuster Video was too focused on its goal of making more money by collecting fines for late rental returns, they didn't accept that the world around them had changed. Netflix on the other hand, free from such a fixed goal, pivoted, they scrapped late fees, instead, they focused on a subscription model. Blockbuster's rigid goals and inflexibility were their demise when the landscape changed whereas Netflix has become one of the biggest entertainment media companies on the planet. Ditching our goals gives us the flexibility to change tack when an opportunity comes along.

I wanted to own a dental practice before I started dental school. I even set myself a goal of owning a practice within ten years of qualifying and there's no doubt I could have done it if ticking that goal off was my only priority. If I'd done so though, I would have had to compromise the development of my clinical skills and give up time from my home life. I started saving with my very first paycheque, but I knew there was still so much to learn about dentistry and business before I would be ready to lead the line. Year after year, I developed my clinical skills and I sought education in business and leadership in dentistry wherever possible. When finally, the ideal opportunity arose, eleven years after I'd qualified, I was ready to take it and I was in a far better place to give it 100% than if I'd jumped in early just for the sake of hitting an arbitrary deadline that I'd set ten years earlier.

## Habits

This might sound strange as you're reading my book, but I'm not a writer. I've always been ungood in English, it was my lowest GCSE grade, probably because I'd hardly read a book until I was nearly 30. I started writing in July 2019 by noting one line a day as a personal journal. This momentary reflection before bed could be something significant that had happened that day, how I was feeling at that moment, an interesting quote or just something funny one of the kids had said. Still, I often found it difficult to think of what to write, it would take me ten minutes to think of five words. Like implementing any new habit, it stuck when I made it easy. I set a reminder on my phone for every evening and kept each entry short and simple. After a while, I found that one line wasn't enough, so I wrote two, then five, and then however many lines it took for me to express my feelings about the day.

I started writing my aspirations for the day in the morning and I realised that other people may benefit from reading my musings, particularly about mental health which is where my blog began. Everyone says it's ok to talk, but very few people actually seemed to do so, I wanted to buck that trend. The more I wrote, the more cathartic it became and the more I realised that I could use my writing to inspire people. In 2020, when a fellow implant dentist Ferhan Ahmed told me he was writing a book, Being Unstoppable, he watered the seeds I'd already planted for me to do the same. I hadn't started writing with the intention of writing a book, that destination wasn't even on my map. I wanted to improve my ability to reflect and appreciate the day and because I'd made the habit easy to begin with, it stuck and it blossomed. One little habit done for the reward of the process, not the outcome has led me way beyond what I'd have done had I set myself a goal of keeping a diary for a month.

James Clear's book, Atomic Habits, teaches the compounding benefits of positive habits. By making a small and sustainable improvement every day we can grow far beyond the sum of the parts. A 1%

improvement each day amounts to a 37-fold improvement in a single year. There are no sensational breakthrough moments, no quick hit of dopamine, only sustainable progress, made minute by minute, hour by hour, day by day. If we focus on making just one tiny change at a time, we're far more likely to make it stick than if we attempt a seismic overhaul which becomes impossible to maintain in the long term. By making these small changes, these habits, every day, we can radically improve not just our clinical skills but also our physical and mental wellbeing.

"We are what we consistently do. Excellence therefore, is not an act, but a habit."
**Aristotle**

Five years after uni, I left the predominantly NHS positions I'd had since foundation training to move to Yorkshire. When I accepted a job at Lindley Dental in Huddersfield, I realised that 95% of my work would be private and I was nervous, I was an NHS dentist and I was now expected to provide private dental care. I felt exposed and vulnerable, like being catapulted back to high school when at any moment I might get busted for pretending to be 'normal' like everyone else when I knew I didn't fit in. I needed to improve, to justify absconding from the NHS, but I also realised that I couldn't change everything in one go.

My first small change was to upgrade my check-ups to dental health reviews. A check-up is tick-boxing to get patients through their pass or fail examination as quickly as possible. A dental health review is actively listening to my patient before conducting a comprehensive assessment of a patient's presenting condition, oral cancer status, temporomandibular joint health, oral hygiene, tooth surface loss, periodontal condition, caries presence and risk assessments. It began though, simply by changing the name and in doing so, changing my mindset about what I was doing. It's a bad idea to try and change everything at once. If we keep the steps small and simple, we make it easy to keep stepping forwards, getting a little better every day.

If day one was about changing the name, day two might mean that instead of trying to get my patient horizontal as quickly as I could, I would ask every patient if they were happy with their teeth. This deliberately open and vague question allows my patients to talk about what is important to them, whether it's related to the health of their teeth or their appearance. Not only am I allowing my patients to give me more information to help them, but I'm also showing them that I care about them as a person, not just what's going on in their mouth.

With each new day comes the opportunity to implement another new habit or stamp out a bad one. The easier a habit is to implement, the easier it is to maintain. These habits don't need to be clinical, in fact, it's vital to implement non-clinical habits. Habits can include exercising before work every day, making sure you arrive on site 30 minutes before your first patient, eating fruit instead of crisps at lunch, and anything that will make your life a little better, one tiny step at a time. These easy to maintain little tweaks incrementally improve our practice and our lives, day by day.

Find your habits by asking yourself these questions:

1. What steps can I take today that will put me in a better position in the future?
2. What can I improve that will enhance my patient experience?
3. What do the best professionals do every day that I don't do?

# Make It Easy

Once you've got some answers, break them down into small, easy to implement steps that you can start doing straight away. Then start, one step at a time, day in, day out. It is imperative that you don't try to implement too much in one go. If a new habit involves a big change, it's going to be much harder to maintain and so by breaking things down into bitesize chunks, they become much easier to implement and sustain.

Breaking bad habits is just as important as starting good ones. It follows that if we can stick to a new habit by making it easy, we break bad habits by making them hard. For a time, I found myself drawn to Facebook on my phone when I had a gap between patients. It became a problem when I was getting so distracted that patients would arrive and I wouldn't notice, I'd keep them waiting until my nurse rightly kicked me. The solution, don't bring my phone onto clinic. I rarely need my phone while I'm seeing patients and even though at first, when I'd get a gap I'd think of flicking onto my socials, my phone was out of reach, so I just didn't do it.

We can also make good habits harder to break by engaging the people around us. By telling our friends and colleagues about the changes we're making, we give ourselves a moral contract that we feel obliged to stick to, lest we let ourselves down in the eyes of those around us. Our colleagues can be invaluable in keeping us on the right track once they know what and why we're doing things. I arrived at work one morning several years ago, following a particularly inspiring talk about bonding, and announced that from that point on, I was going to use the rubber dam for every restoration I did. I told them why; reducing debris in the patient's mouth, better isolation for placing restorations and so on. I had publicly made the commitment and having explained the benefits, my resolve, and asked for their support, everyone was on board. Now, before every restoration, the rubber dam is ready to go and so it's much easier for me to implement the habit. I feel bad if I don't use it because I know they've gone to the effort of getting it ready for me and I'd be breaking my own rules if I skipped it.

We love labelling ourselves and the people around us, we all know people who are the 'clever ones', 'creatives', 'car lovers' or 'fitness fanatics'. We shoehorn everyone into neat little colour-coded personality types in an attempt to simplify a complex world. These labels give us a sense of belonging, sometimes they can drive us forward but often they hold us back. The smoker who's trying to quit is far less likely to succeed than the person who's now labelled themselves as a non-smoker. Do you try and get out for a run three times a week or are you a runner? A bad golfer is always better than someone who tries to play golf.

I said earlier that I'm not a writer but that changed when I decided to write a book. I didn't wait for publication to change my own label. This little shift in mentality to label ourselves as the person we're striving to be will strengthen our resolve to validate the label. It won't make you any better on day one, but it will help you maintain the habits that will help you grow. It might not seem like much, but calling myself a writer gave me the strength I needed on the difficult days when I didn't feel like showing up, to get through it and maintain my writing habit. Ultimately, it's why you're able to read this book today.

## The Pay-Off

There is no immediate pay-off when we start this process, each little change will have very little impact on your life, which is precisely why it works. In a life where everything seems to give us immediate gratification, it's easy to become disillusioned when we can't see tangible benefits straight away. This becomes particularly apparent when we hit roadblocks, those negative events that make us question ourselves, things like a missed diagnosis, seeing our work fail or an unhappy patient. These things happen to every dentist and it's important that we keep focusing on the process of learning and improving, not the blips that these negative outcomes are. We must continue to build our good habits every day, habits that will keep helping us for the rest of our careers until the day comes when we may be able to look back and see how far we've come. Constantly improving by implementing new habits every day is not easy, but it's because it is hard that it's worth doing.

"It never gets easier, you just go faster."
**Greg LeMond**

When you work out in the gym, you put your muscles under stress, as you keep pushing, they start to fatigue, the pain kicks in, your body's saying no but you push yourself to do one more rep. It hurts, but it's that last rep that means you'll come back stronger next time. Growing isn't easy, each new habit will guide you to be a little bit better, stretching your capabilities and pushing you out of your comfort zone.

The aim is to nudge forward just enough every day to grow a little stronger. When something becomes easy, it's no longer helping us to grow and it's at this point we need to add in another small habit to make it that bit more difficult again. By keeping our habits small and easy to implement, we can stress our bodies and minds just enough to continually grow, without the risk of burning out by taking on too much too soon.

There will of course come a day when you miss a habit, you decide to skip the rubber dam because you're running behind and it's only a little cavity anyway. It happens. Sometimes we fall back into an old bad habit too. The sooner we get back on track, the easier it is to keep moving forward. Chastising ourselves for slipping up on one day doesn't help, but getting back on it as soon as possible does. We must try to maintain the momentum we've built through our compounded habits. If we miss a habit on one day, we need to double down to make sure we do it on the next.

"Missing once is an accident. Missing twice is the start of a new habit."
**James Clear**

Finally, our willpower is weakest towards the end of the day, when we're mentally drained from the 35,000 decisions we've already had to make. Habits are easier to stick to when we try to implement them at the start of the day, though just knowing about this willpower fatigue can provide the self-awareness to not be defeated as the day draws to a close.

# Coda

| Three steps to mastery |
|---|
| 1.  Use the questions on page 48 to help you identify where you can improve your work and life. |
| 2.  Break these changes down into their smallest possible components. |
| 3.  Implement these habits one day at a time, engaging the people around you and making them as easy as possible to maintain. |

We do not need a list of arbitrary targets to push ourselves forward. By focusing on our purpose and using this to guide our direction we can do away with goals and implement daily habits that will improve our process. Doing so will sustainably lay the foundations for a fulfilling career. It takes patience and discipline to remove the urge for immediate gratification, but by focusing on the process and not the outcomes we will far surpass any goals we would have set.

When COVID hit, any goals about growing my implant practice would have gone out the window. Instead of blaming misfortune for stopping me from hitting my targets, I pivoted, implementing a new habit of asking every patient with a denture or a gap if they're happy, or if they'd rather have a fixed tooth that will allow them to smile confidently and start to enjoy their food again. I also made sure that at the end of every patient's journey, they were happy and I'd ask them if they'd be willing to recommend me to their friends and family. By implementing these habits and acting on them for every patient, my implant practice has grown organically and I'm in a much better position now than if I had started setting arbitrary targets. In the first couple of years, I may have done less than 50 implants, but the long-term growth is far stronger and shows no signs of abating.

Make your good habits easy and your bad habits hard, and make a pledge to your colleagues so they can help and hold you accountable. Don't be afraid to give yourself a label that will allow you to embody the change you want to become. By slowly building our good habits and eliminating our bad ones, day by day, we will make meaningful changes to our work and life, changes that stick because we've built them up gradually and made them easy to maintain.

By focusing on the parts of our life that we can control we will reap the compounding benefits of our habits, making us more effective in our daily life without distracting from the bigger picture. By accepting that it's not easy, we can forgive our lapses and maintain our momentum by getting back on it the next day. When we encounter obstacles on our path, we will be better equipped to deal with them and when an opportunity comes along, we'll be ready to take it.

# 4

# Lucky Man

## The Verve

### *How to find and take opportunities*

"Chance favours the prepared mind."
**Louis Pasteur**

Adversity takes many forms and I'm very aware that as a straight white male in the UK, I've been given a great number of opportunities and faced fewer barriers in my life than many people reading this book. What I still have to this day though, is the face of a ten year old. I have always looked young and for years this upset me. Being told that I'll be glad of it when I'm older never helped me build confidence with a patient who thinks I'm the work experience kid.

When I graduated, I had just turned 23. In my foundation year, I was bombarded daily with comments about my age or more accurately, my perceived age, which varied between nine and thirteen. I began feeling that my ineradicably immature mug, still devoid of facial hair, undermined all the countless hours of study I'd put into getting where I was. My foundation trainer took great joy in recounting the time a patient asked him 'does his mother know he's out?' Or the countless times he had to reassure patients 'yes, honestly, he is a real dentist.' There were many times the patient would come into the room and with a wry smile look over to the dental nurse as if to say, 'this is some kind of joke, right?'

I felt undermined and under-respected for my achievements. I constantly had to justify my presence, to reassure them that I was a real dentist, pointing to my prominently displayed BDS certificate to prove my worth. This wasn't helped by the foundation dentist preceding being a mature student, nearly twice my age, though no more experienced. I was festooned with a frustration that he never had to deal with, it was assumed, because he looked older, that he was more capable and more qualified. I took a lot of stick in school for looking young and now, in the real world with three big capital letters after my name it continued. I just didn't look like a dentist.

Countless people fear 'the dentist'. Entire populations are haunted by images of a codger in a lab coat by the name of Dr Payne, reeking of a caustic cocktail of TCP and old socks, who would take teeth out without anaesthetic in a sadistic tirade that plagued the community (or so I'm told). I don't have to bear the cross of being associated with that guy. I'm nothing like him, just look at me. And so, I told my patients this, I made this my USP. Every day, they'd come in and tell me their Kubrickian nightmares and I'd listen and reassure them. I'd tell them 'I probably don't look like any other dentist you've seen before' and with that simple statement of the obvious, they'd know this was going to be different. Perhaps it was that I was willing to be patient, listen and acknowledge their angst before I spoke, but every time I'd have the same reaction, the patient would relax and open up about how they really felt about their teeth.

"Responsibility is the ability to choose your response."
**Stephen Covey**

Learning to accept the things I can't change, like looking young, allowed me to see past the problem to find a solution. There are many things in life that we can do nothing about, but what we can do, is choose how we're going to react to them. We can feel held back by our working environment, relationships or a lack of opportunity but looking for someone to blame won't help us grow, we can only play the cards we're dealt. By focusing our energies on the things we can control, we can begin to make meaningful changes. A bad situation never gets better by ignoring it and if a good situation is allowed to pass us by, we may miss an opportunity to maximise its potential. For years I tried to ignore the fact that I looked young but it didn't change anything, it was only by confronting it head-on that I was able to take responsibility for my situation and choose a response that made my baby face work to my advantage.

# Opportunities

There is never a perfect time to take the next leap into the unknown, whether it's a step forward in our professional career or personal life. Opportunities don't present themselves at ideal times either, in fact, to say they present themselves at all is a misnomer. The dream job in a great practice may become available before you feel ready to take that leap. You may feel like you're not worthy of the position, or you don't have the skills that you feel someone in that position should have.

I certainly felt like this when I took my first job in a mostly private practice. I questioned whether I was good enough technically as a dentist to provide a private level of treatment. The opportunity of a job in a private practice for me came about because of the lack of good opportunities in independent NHS practices. I went for interviews at two private practices and was offered the job at both. I realised that if these principal dentists who had worked for years in private practice thought I was good enough to care for their patients in their practices, then the issue of my skill level was probably more in my own head. The reality I can see now is that I would never have felt completely ready to take that step. You never become competent at something before you start doing it.

Opportunities surround us all the time, yet we frequently fail to see them or having seen them, we let them pass by. Early in our careers, it helps to take advantage of as many opportunities as possible. When you start looking you will find opportunities that you're not ready for and that's fine. It's better to identify too many, even if you're not ready for some than to be completely unaware of any potential opportunities. The greater awareness you have of the available opportunities, the better you'll be able to identify the unmissable ones.

We have three valuable tools to cultivate opportunities; education, communication and diversification.

## Education

Education is the first and simplest step to take in preparing ourselves for new opportunities. The more knowledge we have on a subject, the more confident we will feel in taking the next step forward. Of course, it takes time and dedication to develop the knowledge and skills to become a competent general dentist and it would be reckless to try and jump too many steps without laying the appropriate foundations. However, there will never be a time when it feels comfortable taking that leap of faith and that's great news because you never know when the right opportunity is going to arise. All we can do is prepare ourselves by maximising our knowledge before an opportunity comes and goes.

## Communication

The best opportunities will come about through the people we already know, maybe not directly, but within one degree of separation. Dunbar's number suggests that we're able to maintain 150 social relationships at any one time. This is 150 people who may be able to help us find a great new opportunity or a staggering 22,500 people who are just one connection away from us. Social media allows us to connect with thousands of people, but this doesn't mean we can vouch for their personality, morals or skills in the way that knowing someone in the real world can. By nurturing a broad network, not necessarily with more people but a diverse group, we can often help connect like-minded individuals in disparate careers and in turn, we may discover opportunities for ourselves in the most unlikely places.

Diversification

We can maximise the number of opportunities we find by keeping a diverse range of interests inside and outside of dentistry. By building a range of skills, some that often seem completely unrelated to our clinical work, we can uncover hidden talents, develop different ways of thinking and find new passions. It's this diversity in our skillset that will help us when we reflect to recalibrate our direction moving forward.

A diverse range of skills also liberates us from the danger of losing everything in one fell swoop. If we keep all our eggs in one basket, dropping that basket is a disaster. If you've got your eggs spread across five baskets, dropping one is an inconvenience. I worked across three practices in my first few years after foundation training and this meant that when the relationship with the principal dentist at one practice broke down, I could move on despite not having anywhere specific to move to. There were times, for sure, when I wanted to get comfortable in one room, with one nurse and not be travelling around all the time, but the inconvenience was a trade-off for better long-term prospects.

I began my career by laying the foundations of knowledge in the subjects I was fascinated by. I've maintained a blend of different jobs in a variety of settings, alongside mentoring, lecturing and now writing, all of which have allowed me to connect with a broad group of people. Doing so has not only kept my work interesting with its variety but I've also given myself some security that if one job goes awry, I have other positions to fall back on. I'm also in the best place to seek out new opportunities and in an ideal position to take them.

No opportunity is ever perfect, a new job is always a slightly bigger commute, not quite the perfect hours or comes with a degree of risk or uncertainty. There's always a hitch and having a neurotic personality and a perfectionist attitude, which most dentists do, we can easily justify our decision not to take an opportunity. This neuroticism can help us to focus on the minutiae which is important for much of our work, from caries removal to soft tissue surgery. This can be a useful trait but neurotics are rarely relaxed, we stress and we zoom in on the details, infatuated by whatever's in the narrow field of view of our shiny new 7.5x mag refractive loupes. We often fail to see the bigger picture and this loss of perspective inhibits our ability to spot opportunities as they develop. If you've never done it before, now is a good time to stop reading and watch Daniel Simons' selective attention test, the one where you have to count the number of passes the team in white makes....

Did you see it? There are many forms of this test, but the point is the same, when you focus on the specifics, you fail to see the bigger picture. When I graduated, I decided it was time to upgrade my little Vauxhall Corsa to the Alfa Romeo Giulietta. Not just any Giulietta though, the 1.4 litre multi-air engine, manual gearbox, in Etna Black, with cruise control and heated seats. I couldn't afford a brand new one but I wanted it in like-new condition with low mileage and well within warranty. Being so specific made it near impossible to find the right one, every time a car came available there was something not quite right, by the time I'd decided I'd been too specific, the second and third best alternatives had already gone. When the right car finally came along, I had to pay over the odds to make sure I got it. In waiting for the perfect car, I'd missed several opportunities to get a great car and wasted a lot more time, energy and money.

If we wait for perfection, we're going to be waiting a long time. At the time I cursed my bad luck because the car I wanted wasn't available, without realising that by finding fault with everything, the problem wasn't the cars, but me. I thought it was bad luck that meant I wasn't driving the car I wanted when really, luck had nothing to do with it.

# Luck

What we perceive as luck in everyday life often has far more to do with mindset and preparation than pure chance. Was Alexander Fleming lucky when he returned from his jollies in 1928 and found an accumulation of mould in a petri dish? This mould, formed from the remnants of his lunch before his vacation, had stopped the proliferation of a sample of Staphylococci. He christened this magical mould, Penicillin. How many busy professors would have missed this, cleaning away the old dishes without a second glance to make way for the next experiment? How many would have seen the mould and reasoned it away using erroneous preconceptions? Fleming's discovery was only made possible by his years of experience in the field of microbiology and his persistently inquisitive and observant nature. His openness to his own ignorance and his readiness to spot new opportunities resulted in modern medicine's greatest 'lucky' discovery.

You will often find the greatest achievers attributing much of their success to luck and it's precisely because they consider themselves lucky that they can identify the opportunities around them. If you took part in one of Professor Richard Wiseman's studies, after filling out your luck profile questionnaire to establish how lucky or unlucky you feel you are, you would be asked to go to a coffee shop and get yourself a coffee. What you wouldn't be told, is that they'd planted a £5 note right outside the door. The results showed that more often than not, the people who considered themselves lucky found themselves £5 richer and the unlucky ones walked straight past it. People who consider themselves lucky, live with their eyes open, whereas the unlucky in life exist blinkered to the world around them, unable to see or embrace the opportunities that come their way.

> "Being in the right place at the right time is actually all about being in the right state of mind."
> **Richard Wiseman**

We can't think our way to winning the lottery, but we can live in a state where we're ready to embrace luck, where we can spot the opportunities that would otherwise pass us by. Opportunities, like habits, compound, meaning as you take advantage of one opportunity, it's likely to lead to several more. Once the ball starts rolling, you will find a constant stream of opportunities available to you and the problem then becomes less about finding them and more about deciding which ones to take.

## Decision Making

When you've started to take advantage of these opportunities, you will reach a saturation point, a time when you simply can't fit any more in. It's a nice problem to have of course, but it still needs to be dealt with. To overcome this problem you're going to have to ask yourself a difficult question.

Which part of my life am I willing to sacrifice to take the next opportunity?

I've never been willing to cut my family time. I knew I wanted to do more mentoring and lecturing, but it was going to be difficult to fit this around my full-time work schedule. By taking the time to ask myself what I was going to sacrifice before the opportunity arose, I was able to take steps in my life to be ready for the opportunity. In the first instance, this meant having a conversation with my principal dentist about how she'd feel about me taking some time away from my regular clinics to do this. This conversation must happen before the opportunity arises, if it happens after and the answer is a categorical no, then it will take time to find a solution, by the time it is sorted, the opportunity may have passed. By having this conversation early, not only did I put myself in the best position to be ready for the opportunity, but I was being honest with the people who would be affected by my decisions.

The right opportunity is usually the one that will offer a long-term benefit to your life rather than an immediate one. When it comes to a job, this sometimes means a drop in income to gain more experience or travelling further to be in the right environment to thrive. Difficult decisions usually involve consciously entering into a period of discomfort as we move from something we've been doing well, back to the position of the novice. When it comes to making big or even small decisions, I refer back to my purpose and use this to help me find the right answer. Sometimes, taking an opportunity may directly impact my purpose but often it's something that will improve my quality of life in a way that will help me fulfil my purpose indirectly.

If I'm struggling, I use the five-year regret test. Picture yourself in five years in both lives, the first having taken the opportunity, the second having turned it down. Which life is better? Which decision are you more likely to regret? Contextualising our decisions into the bigger picture will make some choices feel completely irrelevant and others quite momentous. Taking the long-term view will also help overcome our subconscious bias towards immediate gratification.

We don't have a crystal ball, but by giving time to consider what's going to put us in the best position in the future based on our purpose, we can maintain our direction without getting sidetracked by short-term gains that won't add value to our lives. The only way to completely lose is not to decide at all. Deciding to say 'no', or even 'not right now' allows everyone to move on.

We have one more tool in our decision-making arsenal, intuition. We are creatures of habit, pattern finders and familiarity seekers and our brains do this subconsciously. This is one of the reasons why making improvements in the form of habits is so effective. Our intuition is the inner voice that tells us when something feels right or wrong based on our past experiences. These experiences have often been relegated to our subconscious, but they're not completely forgotten. Our subconscious recognises patterns and behaviours that we've previously encountered and guides us to the right answer. Intuition can't be solely relied upon, but it often gives us a nudge in the right direction.

We trust our intuition all day, every day, including when diagnosing teeth. During my foundation year, I would jump back and forth in my mind as to whether some fissure staining required intervention. I'd ask my mentor to give me his opinion and he would take one look and tell me how deep the cavity would be. I was amazed at how he would always be right, based on a cursory glance into the patient's mouth. We can't always verbalise how we get to the right answer, but often we know it's right. It's the nuances of each situation that our brains have programmed into our subconscious that allow us to make most of the thousands of decisions we make daily, without having to expend significant mental energy.

We can't trust our intuition with new situations, we've simply not had the experience to make the process subconscious yet, but as our experience grows, we can intuitively find solutions to progressively more complex problems. It's particularly important to trust the inner voice that tells us when something doesn't feel right. This might be whether or not to provide advanced treatment for a patient or if we think our patient has fully understood the treatment we're proposing. In either case, if our gut says 'no', then we'd better take it seriously. The more experience we have in an area, the more reliable our intuition becomes. Diagnosing simple diseases of teeth becomes second nature after a couple of years, we can make most decisions and discuss the best treatment options with little need for the exhausting deliberation that every cavity required in the early days.

Intuition does not replace evidence when making

clinical decisions, but it can guide us in the right direction, particularly outside our oral confines. Just like finding the right opportunities and being lucky, intuition is not something that just happens. Intuition comes about through hard work and dedication. It's about putting ourselves in situations that challenge us and make us do the work in the first place, to train our brains to process information more efficiently and then trust it to do this job.

# Coda

| Three steps to mastery |
|---|
| 1. Education - Arm yourself with the knowledge to be ready for opportunities as they arise. |
| 2. Communication - Nurture a broad network that can help you support others as they may be able to help you. |
| 3. Diversification - Maintain a broad spectrum of interests inside and outside of dentistry, disparate skills and opportunities frequently cross-pollenate. |

Fortune and misfortune are happening around us all the time and you never really know which one is which until you can look back. Breaking my arm during my foundation year felt like misfortune (mixed with stupidity) until I was able to change my perspective and realise that I had been given the gift of time to use in other ways. Looking young has always felt like a curse but again I was able to find a way to make it work for me. We all face challenges on our journey, we will grow strongest by learning to take action on the things we can control and to change our attitude about the things we can't. Progress in life will come more from reframing challenges and identifying opportunities than from luck, but we can prepare ourselves and be ready to embrace the opportunities that come our way.

The perfect opportunity may never come, but by ensuring we have an open mind we can be prepared to embrace any opportunity that will add value to our life. When it comes to choosing the right opportunity to take, our purpose can be our guide and we can be ready to take it if we have already decided what will need to sacrifice to do so.

No matter how powerful our purpose is, how effective our habits are, or how many advantages we can embrace, we will always find obstacles on our path. No matter how positively we try to maintain our mindset, we all have bad days, bad things happen sometimes. Ignoring the warning light on the dashboard doesn't fix the engine and pretending that we live in an entirely positive world will only lead to disappointment when life falls below our expectations. Dentistry can feel like a very unforgiving profession and it presents a unique set of challenges that are often common only to those in healthcare. Facing up to the challenges themselves can be hard enough but it's the persistent fear of them that can completely erode our passion. I want to be prepared for these challenges so I know that when they happen, I can take them in my stride and I don't have to live in fear of them

# 5

# There Goes the Fear

## Doves

### *How to practise without fear*

"The ultimate measure of a man is not where he stands in moments of comfort and convenience but where he stands in times of challenge and controversy."
**Martin Luther King Jr**

I haven't always loved being a dentist. There was a time when the fear of complaints, litigation, regulation and endless bureaucracy would weigh on my mind every moment of every day. They'd be a key factor in deciding which treatment I should provide for a patient, above what was actually best for them. Then there's the pressure I'd put on myself to be perfect, to never make a mistake, to not be human. We can't possibly perform at our best if our minds are plagued with these fears. Not only is it emotionally exhausting, but our clinical decisions tend to be towards what has been dubbed 'defensive dentistry' which often means providing the safest treatment for us, rather than the best treatment for our patients. If we're going to learn, grow, maintain our passion and give our patients the best level of care, we need to overcome these fears.

The first solution is to understand why most problems arise in the first place. Inappropriate expectations are the root cause of many of the issues we face. Either we've failed to meet our patient's expectations or we've failed to live up to the impossible standards we set for ourselves. Happiness is an outcome that is dependent on expectations. If life is better than we expect, we're happy, if it's falling short, we're sad. The same principle is true for our patients, if we meet or exceed their expectations, they're happy, if we fail to do this, they're disappointed. It's an exceedingly simple perspective but one which has huge ramifications for our whole lives.

Our patients all come with preconceived ideas about how their treatment will turn out, what it will look like, how long it will take and how much pain they will have. It is our responsibility to make sure these expectations align with what we believe we can achieve. If we don't think we can meet a patient's expectations before treatment, then it's best not to even start. As my experience has built in dentistry, I find myself being more pessimistic with my patients about the outcomes I can achieve. Outcomes after all are often beyond my control. I'll be clear with my patients that I'm giving them the worst-case scenario but for them to give valid consent, they have to be prepared to face the worst because unfortunately, the worst does happen sometimes.

Patients don't usually become unhappy following a single incident, rather it's the culmination of multiple missed opportunities to put things right. There will often be several small issues, which I call grumbles, that occur every day that we have the opportunity to rectify before things escalate. These grumbles usually emerge in a passing comment from a patient who's otherwise very happy with our care. Rather than smiling and nodding or offering a cursory apology, these comments are listened to and recorded in a grumble book, which is then discussed as a team so we can take steps to prevent the situation from recurring. The problems arise when multiple little grumbles accumulate for a single patient which builds dissatisfaction, which precedes a significant event, resulting in a more serious complaint. By empowering the team to speak up and be involved in finding solutions to the little things, we mitigate the risk of a bigger problem down the line. A stitch in time saves nine.

A patient recently came to me for his dental health review and having arrived late, he'd missed his appointment with our hygienist immediately before. He was upset because he'd been told he'd have to rebook which meant more time out of his busy schedule. He was also frustrated and embarrassed about missing the appointment. Now we could blame our patient, but he'd been at the practice for years and had always had his dental health review first, so he hadn't expected the appointments to be the other way around. By listening, acknowledging the issue and asking the patient how we could avoid this problem happening again, not only did we show him we care, but we could actively start taking steps to prevent other patients from falling foul of the same confusion.

As with nearly all problems that arrive in any relationship, dental or otherwise, miscommunication was at the very heart of the matter. The antidote to miscommunication is always communication.

## Complaints

When a patient makes a formal complaint, as well as the accumulation of grumbles, there are often other precipitating factors such as anxiety, stress, time pressures, financial concerns, or any number of personal factors. These can affect the patient, the clinician, or both and with such a maelstrom of emotion, the greatest challenge is to act rationally. We can take it personally, feeling unjustly persecuted, but any patient who's gone to the trouble of making a formal complaint will feel justified in their actions, however unjust we may feel they're being.

Our immediate response may be to try to defend ourselves and deflect blame onto someone else or even the patient, but this often aggravates the situation. The most important first step is to respond calmly and to try to understand our patient's grievance. If a complaint is made verbally, we must simply listen and ask further questions until we fully understand the root cause of the problem. Reflecting this back to the patient shows them that we've listened and are trying to see things from their perspective. By allowing our patient time to talk and then working with them instead of against them, we can usually find a solution together.

I always prefer to speak in person when there is a grievance, so much of communication is lost in words on a page, though it's customary to respond like-for-like with the chosen method of communication. Written complaints, therefore, can be more awkward to deal with. A prompt response is critical to make sure the patient feels heard, even if it's just to acknowledge receipt. I would speak to my defence organisation on receipt of a written complaint, even if it's just to check my response is appropriate. In principle, the solution remains the same, we must seek first to understand before we try to take action to make the problem go away.

"The opposite of love is not hate, but indifference."
**Wilhelm Stekel**

People don't complain about things they don't care about. If someone cares enough to let you know when things haven't gone as expected, we must take it seriously and embrace the opportunity to make amends. Once our patient sees that we care and that we want to work with them, not against them, we can find a solution before problems escalate.

# Litigation

We don't always have the luxury of being able to talk to our patients before the leaden letter lands.

*15th June*

*This evening I had a phone call from my former principal dentist, he's received a letter from a solicitor on behalf of a patient who I'd done a few fillings for a few years ago. Jess came to me to check her teeth before travelling abroad for several months. I found a few holes but she didn't come back to get them all fixed before leaving the country. When she returned, I filled the now bigger holes which lead to some post-operative pain and two teeth ultimately required root canal treatment. I remember Jess because we got on well, we'd chatted about where she was going and I enjoyed catching up with her adventures when she returned.*

*When she started having issues after my treatment, I'd taken the time to explain why and I thought we'd cleared things up. That was the last I heard from her until today when the letter arrived. I'm always upset when one of my patients has pain, especially following treatment I've provided. I'm also upset that I didn't get the opportunity to put things right for her and I feel betrayed by someone who I'd got on well with.*

Whilst part of me felt unfairly attacked, I questioned my clinical abilities and my communication skills. I was no longer sure if I was in the right job and whether dentistry was worth the stress and fear of this litigation. This was at a time when I felt I had acquired a reasonable level of skills as a general dentist and it destroyed my confidence. I questioned everything I was doing for every patient, every hour of every day, for weeks on end. I would also be starkly aware of the threat of another solicitor's letter with every clinical interaction I would make.

*2nd July*

*As I lay in bed, Marisa says I've been distracted for the past few weeks, I've not been my normal self. I've been trying to give my full attention to my family but I know I'm stressed, I think about the solicitor's letter every day and I'm finding it hard to concentrate on anything else.*

*After the initial shock and worry, I've had numerous extremely positive interactions with other patients. Superficially I feel better but my confidence is low, my trust in others diminished and I have this persistent feeling of vulnerability.*

*12th July*

*I've had to wear my bite guard for the past few weeks, I haven't been sleeping great and I'm overwhelmed by a feeling of apathy. I feel like a black hole, sucking the life out of those closest to me.*

Reading this back now, whilst it feels dramatic, it reflects how I felt at the time. I realise that I'm fortunate not to have a story to tell where things progressed further and many may scoff at the protracted drama that played out in my mind over something that never got beyond first base. That said, it still hurt. I felt vulnerable, I felt attacked and it affected me deeply.

I don't remember when it stopped playing on my mind every day and the advice from my indemnifier wasn't in any way compassionate or reassuring. I was told I just had to submit my clinical notes and wait and see. What happened next was, as it turns out, absolutely nothing. No further correspondence from the patient or the solicitor.

My hugely simplified understanding of what happens in these cases is that the notes get sent to an 'expert' dentist who knows all the answers to what is right and wrong in every situation. This expert peruses the notes and gives the solicitor an opinion as to whether they think the accused dentist has done anything wrong. My best guess is that the expert looked at my notes and decided they were good enough to make it more hard work than it was worth to pursue litigation.

"He who suffers before it is necessary, suffers more than it is necessary."
**Lucius Annaeus Seneca**

Through this experience, the mental summersaults and the eventual acceptance of the climate we live in, I've come to a few conclusions:

1.  I will always try to do my best for my patients and I can't do this if I'm living in fear of reprimand. I will continually learn and try to improve my skills to

better help my patients and if I can do this, I can sleep well.

2.  I will always keep the best possible clinical records, record every diagnosis, document every conversation and log every action taken or refused. If or when it goes wrong, they may just save me a whole lot of hassle.

3.  I will build open and trusting relationships with all my patients, I will trust them and that they, in turn, will trust me. I will not punish the thousands of wonderful patients that I'm privileged to be able to help for the fear that one person may betray my trust.

# Regulation

It's essential that we have a well regulated profession to protect patients from harm by that very, very small minority of clinicians who don't practice ethically. Regulation shouldn't exist to scare the daylights out of honest, hardworking clinicians but to help us maintain public trust and respect for the profession. I remember the fear of God being put into me as an undergraduate about the people who could end my career and that they probably would, given any opportunity. A time when having received a complaint, it would take two years to establish whether or not your entire life and livelihood would be torn apart, often before deciding to drop the case as soon as someone with a rational head looked at it and realised it was nonsense.

Times are changing though. Cases are being processed

more quickly if they even get that far in the first place. Patients are encouraged to raise grievances directly with their dental practice and only consider escalating the most serious issues that could cause significant harm to the public. There are three criteria used to assess whether someone is safe to continue to practise:

1. Insight - do you understand that a mistake was made and how it happened?
2. Remediation - have you told the patient and taken appropriate steps to put it right?
3. Repetition - have you made this same mistake repeatedly, or are you likely to?

Knowing this, our solution is simple, we must accept that we're not perfect, acknowledge when we make a mistake and take steps to prevent it from happening again. Take these simple steps and we have no reason to fear regulation.

We can't provide our best care if we're working in fear of litigation and regulation. 'Defensive dentistry' is not providing the best care for our patients. I have learned to live and work without fear of these external threats and I know I'm providing better care for this. It's the internal battle that has raged on for longer though. The expectation I set of myself to be perfect and the self-flagellation when I make a mistake have been more difficult to overcome.

# Mistakes

"The only real mistake is the one from which we learn nothing."
**Henry Ford**

In the mid-nineteenth century, women all over the world were dying following childbirth of Puerperal fever, a mysterious postpartum disease causing catastrophic organ failure in 25% of new mothers in hospitals. Doctors would spend half their time on the wards bringing new lives into the world and the other half in the morgue performing autopsies, desperately trying to figure out why so many women were dying. It was Doctor Ignaz Semmelweis, working in Vienna hospital, who postulated that it was the very doctors who were frantically searching for the cause of this epidemic who were unwittingly carrying millions of pathogens from the morgue on their unwashed hands back to the next poor mother to be. Unfortunately, doctors didn't take kindly to being told that they were the reason these mothers were dying and so the cycle went on. The mother dies, the doctor performs an autopsy and then carries pathogenic bacteria straight back onto the ward to infect again.

Dr Semmelweis had correctly observed that by implementing mandatory hand washing for doctors, interrupting the bacterial mass transit system, the mortality rate plummeted. Despite demonstrating how this simple hygiene practice could save so many lives, most doctors refused to change their ways, not through malice, but incongruence. They refused to accept their mistake, calling it an insult to implicate that a gentleman would have unclean hands. It took until the latter part of the nineteenth century and the work of Louis Pasteur (he of Pasteurisation) and Robert Koch who disseminated the germ theory of disease, for people outside of Semmelweis's hospital to take notice and introduce what we now consider basic hygiene practices.

There are many failings to learn from this tragic story. Handwashing may seem obvious now, but it was a radical idea at the time and the majority of doctors failed to accept that they could be making a mistake. To this day, we healthcare professionals persecute ourselves with this ideology of perfection, that we should never make a mistake and not only is this unrealistic but it's dangerous.

"I never lose. I either win or learn."
**Nelson Mandela**

When we ignore our mistakes or pretend that we don't make any, we fail to learn and we miss an opportunity to grow. We are human. We all make mistakes. I'm not ashamed to admit that there's not a single day that goes by where I don't think I could have done something a little better. Most of the time, they're minor things that cause no harm, but from time to time I make a more significant mistake. I've caught a patient's cheek with a high speed handpiece, fractured files in root canals, placed restorations that have fallen out and implants that haven't integrated.

When these things happen, I kick myself, I've failed to

meet my own impossible expectations of perfection. I want to do the best possible at all times and when I fall short, it hurts, yet as humans, we will always fall short of perfection. Sometimes I immediately know what I did wrong, other times it's easier to blame misfortune, circumstance, or my patient. Each time something like this happens though, I've reflected, learned and tried to improve things so it doesn't happen again.

Coping with our fallibility is a delicate balance between accepting that as humans we will make mistakes and taking ownership of the issue when something does occur, even in situations when there are multiple factors at work. I can blame a patient for moving while I'm treating them, for instance, but I could have protected their soft tissues better. It's not about apportioning blame to ourselves or anyone else but taking responsibility for the situation. In these unfortunate situations, when something has gone wrong and it's negatively affected the care we've provided, we must be honest with our patients. You will feel vulnerable when admitting an error, but not only is it our duty to be honest, in my experience, patients are far more likely to respect our honesty and these instances often serve to strengthen a relationship.

We all want to do our best for our patients, we always act with the best of intentions and never recklessly or too far beyond our capabilities, so it can be soul-destroying when we feel as though someone has come to harm at our hands. I used to love watching Scrubs, an American comedy-drama that follows a young doctor called JD who idolises his cruelly sarcastic and sadistic mentor, Dr Cox.

In an episode called My Fallen Idol, stressed by the increasing demands on him in a busy hospital, Dr Cox makes a clinical decision that results in the death of three patients. Distraught, he descends into a deep depression which nobody seems to be able to help him out of. JD struggles to come to terms with the fact that his hero isn't actually infallible. On realising the absurdity of this notion, JD eventually goes to his implacable mentor and says 'I came over here to tell you how proud of you I am. Not because you did the best you could for those patients, but because after 20 years of being a doctor, when things go badly, you still take it this hard. And I gotta tell you, man, I mean, that's the kind of doctor I want to be.'

When things don't go according to plan it hurts, all the more so because we care deeply about our patients. Working in fear of making mistakes will lead to us making decisions about what care we provide that appear the simplest and not necessarily what is best. To overcome this, we must be ready to accept that things do go wrong sometimes and having an awareness of when the risks are higher, will help us practice in the safest possible way. We can make mistakes at any time, but they happen more often when we're stressed, fatigued, anxious or when we're working outside of our comfort zone.

Dr James Reason's Swiss cheese model of human factors uses slices of the perforated cheese to symbolise barriers that can prevent a hazard from causing harm. In the dental setting, these hazards are sharps injuries, iatrogenic trauma or mistakes like taking the wrong tooth out, amongst an unquantifiable number of other things. Our barriers are things like appropriate treatment planning, adequate training, mentoring, good communication, using pre-operative checklists and stress management. Each barrier has holes in it, but by lining them all up we reduce the risk of a hazard making it through everyone.

We don't always have complete control over the whole situation, but with an awareness of the hazards and our barriers, we can mitigate the risks. When stepping outside our comfort zone for instance, we know we're going to feel stressed, so we can double down on our planning, make sure we've had appropriate training and communicate clearly with the team around us. These things won't eliminate the risk, but we can grow and practice knowing we've taken steps to provide care in the safest way possible.

# Coda

| Three steps to mastery |
|---|
| 1. Start a grumble book so you can address the small issues before they add up to big ones. Engage the team around you to get more honest feedback. |
| 2. Don't let the fear of litigation and regulation stop you from giving your best care to the people who deserve it. |
| 3. Be human. Accept that we all make mistakes and with this acceptance, learn, improve and minimise the likelihood of them recurring. |

Fear has the potential to suck the passion out of our careers. To be the best professionals we can be, we have to grow beyond fearing these perceived threats and find a way to use all our experiences, positive and negative, to learn and grow. Mistakes happen and we must accept this to be able to mitigate the risk of repeating them. The advice given to me by Professor Simon Wright, my mentor in my foundation year (and for many years since), was 'as long as you always try your best for your patients, no matter what happens, you can hold your head high and sleep well at night.'

Once you have overcome the fear, you're ready to start practising with passion, pushing yourself to the next level to begin to live your purpose. We, of course, want to strive to be the best we can be, but what does it take to perform at our best consistently?

# 6

# Bring It on

## Gomez

### *How to supercharge your growth*

"Whether you believe you can or you can't, you're right."
**Henry Ford**

As a dentist, having a face like a 10 year old immediately lead people to question my level of experience. I realised early on that my patients needed to feel confident in me and I had to do everything I could to enable this. I learned to act more confidently so that I could help my patients better. After a while a strange thing started to happen, the more I acted confident for my patients, the more confident I felt. What started as a pretence, became practice, which became reality. This effect isn't limited to confidence, we become the virtues and values we enact every day.

In order to do anything well, we must approach it with confidence, applying the knowledge and skills we've acquired with conviction and being brave enough to step out of our comfort zone at the right time and with the right support around us. Persistently seeking out new challenges is hard, we need self-confidence to keep moving forward and we need a positive mindset that empowers us to continue when the difficult times come. Doing anything of significance is hard, if it wasn't, everyone would be doing it and if everyone's doing it, it would no longer be significant.

"We choose to go to the moon, not because it is easy, but because it is hard."
**John F Kennedy**

Taking a step outside our comfort zone is, by definition, uncomfortable. It is completely normal to feel anxious when doing anything for the first time. The adrenaline and cortisol coursing through our arteries are preparing our body for fight or flight. These hormones give us the energy to take on the challenges ahead of us, whether that's escaping a predator or placing a dental implant. Pre-performance anxiety is completely normal and if we can identify it, we can own it and use our body's resources to perform at our best.

Owning our feelings in these situations means understanding whether it's caused by a self-imposed fear of inadequacy, or a genuine knowledge that you aren't adequately prepared to undertake the procedure. Either is ok, the first step in remedying the situation is to identify it and accept it. Sometimes, accepting these feelings is enough, other times, this is the trigger for us to seek further support or education before we move forward.

When I was placing my first dental implant, despite the training and the close supervision of my mentor, I was extremely anxious. I was numbing my patient up and my hand was shaking almost as much as it was the first time I gave an ID block in dental school when the tutor had to come over and quite literally hold my hand to keep it steady. Part of my anxiety at that moment, on top of feeling out of my comfort zone, was a feeling that I had to reassure my patient with a facade of confidence. The more I tried to pretend I had everything under control, the harder it became to concentrate on the surgery I was about to perform.

In that moment, I decided to tell my patient this was my first dental implant placement. I should have done this long before, of course. I reassured her (and myself) that I had done the appropriate training and I had the guidance of a mentor alongside me the whole time. She smiled knowingly and said 'we all have to do the first one sometime.' I immediately felt more relaxed. I didn't need to carry the burden of pretending and this allowed me to focus my energy on the procedure itself. If I was unsure about something, I could stop and ask my mentor without fear that the patient would suddenly lose all confidence in me.

When we do anything for the first time, we need to be able to concentrate fully on the procedure itself. We can only do this with a patient who we have a positive, trusting relationship with and this depends entirely on us being honest with our patients about our level of experience. Since the day of my first implant placement, I've always made sure to tell my patient when I'm doing a procedure for the first time, though now I make sure I do it long before I'm about to start their treatment. I've also never had a patient tell me that they don't want me to provide their treatment after being honest about my lack of experience.

# Overconfidence

As my confidence grew, I can see that in time I started to overcompensate. This facade of confidence started to tend towards arrogance. I thought I knew everything I needed to know to be a top dentist already and I just needed a bit more practice. When we're young, we feel invincible, this is why teenagers have such high rates of car crashes. When we're inexperienced, we don't realise how little we know, how poorly we have mastered our craft, whether it's driving or dentistry, and how dangerous this misplaced confidence can be to ourselves and those around us. This isn't a problem restricted to the young, of course, 90% of all drivers think they're better than average, which mathematically, cannot be possible.

At its worst, my arrogance lead me down a path where I was no longer trying to do my best, I was trying to be *the* best. Despite what the awards ceremonies may lead us to feel, we are not in competition in dentistry. Healthcare is not a zero-sum game with winners and losers. There is no grand championship where there will be a single winning dentist that everyone must aspire to be. There is no point when we will be able to say we've completed dentistry either, finished all the levels, defeated the evil professor boss and won the game. The game, if we can call it that, is an infinite one, where the aim is to keep playing for as long as you want to and get a little bit better with each day that passes. One in which we can help to raise others around us without detriment to ourselves so we can all provide our best care for our patients.

There's a delicate balance to be struck between confidence and arrogance and I know I don't always get this right. I need confidence in myself to stride forwards, I need to imbue my patients with this confidence and to some extent, this will always be an act. As I learn more, I discover so many more things that I don't know. How can I have complete confidence in myself when I know there's so much that I don't know? Imposter syndrome often strikes whenever I step out of my comfort zone, when I'm giving a lecture or when something doesn't go according to plan. In these moments, it's reflecting on my successes and reminding myself of my purpose that often helps me through and gives me renewed strength to keep getting better.

When we continually set the bar higher for ourselves, we are deliberately making things difficult and it is confidence that allows us to keep working through these difficult times. Most people quit when things become difficult, when the initial buzz of starting an exciting new path has worn off and all the challenges form a chasm between where we are and where we think we need to get to. This is the worst possible time to stop. We've already committed significant time and energy to this path and quitting at this point means it's all for nothing. When we commit ourselves to a journey, we have to do so with the knowledge that it is going to get hard, and we have to be willing to go through those hardships from the outset. We can quit because we realise we're on the wrong path, but we must not quit because things have become difficult.

Confidence in our abilities alongside our purpose will drive us forward and we can derive positivity from knowing that the difficult times will make us stronger. When we're prepared for the difficult times, we can focus on our process and not our outcomes, and doing so will help us grow regardless of the final result. Life doesn't always go according to plan, but if we've consistently built good habits, we can have faith in our ability to come out the other side of whatever comes our way, whether it's the challenges we've set ourselves or the ones imposed upon us. Confidence in our ability comes through dedicated learning, practice and reflection through the good and the bad. Harnessing this confidence allows us to keep growing.

## Upskilling

Four years after I qualified, I was working in a practice on the Wirral with a foundation dentist, Chirag Patel, Chiggs. If his mentor wasn't available when he needed a hand, I'd do what I could to help him, usually with a tricky extraction, not that he ever needed much help.

What struck me about Chiggs was the exceptional artistry in his work, particularly his composite restorations. He was so much better than me already and he'd barely left dental school. I became disheartened and my confidence took a beating. I had thought I was doing pretty well, I mean, I usually got the shade match roughly right, yet here was this dentist, with so much less experience in the real world, doing these stunning restorations that looked and functioned like natural teeth.

I figured he was just naturally talented. I'd resigned myself to the fact that he was just genetically better than me and there was nothing I could do about it. That was until one lunchtime, I peeled my eyes away from my phone for five minutes and went looking for him. Why hadn't he joined the rest of us during dinner? I found him messing about with a pristine-looking extracted tooth, he'd obviously spent a while getting it clean to practise on. He asked me to see if I could find the filling that he'd just done in it. I couldn't find it. It looked like a perfectly healthy tooth, so much so that I started to question why it had been taken out. It was only then that I realised the whole tooth was made out of composite, with layered shades, tints and glorious root morphology. I realised that while I was playing on my phone, he was spending hour upon hour in deliberate practice, buying himself new gear, investing in himself to get better. I know Chiggs has got some artistic talent in him, but it's the skill that he's dedicated time to developing that makes him exceptional.

We all have unique abilities, some people have a naturally higher level of fitness, and others have better hand-eye coordination but in the real world of everyday dentistry, these differences are practically inconsequential. These natural abilities are discernible in elite sports, where a marginal gain in stamina or agility can make a significant difference at the highest level, but these marginal differences are imperceptible in our profession. Anyone who has sufficient motor skills and acumen to make it through dental school can learn what it takes to provide excellent healthcare.

Nobody is born with the ability to do a perfect crown prep, plan a complex rehabilitation or communicate clearly and confidently with a patient. Natural talent is overrated, skills are not. Skills are the techniques and abilities you acquire through learning and practice. When you see a beautiful case presented, it's not been done with natural talent, it's the same set of skills that anyone can master.

Genetically, we are 99.9% identical to all other humans on the planet. Natural talent can only be a very small part of the remaining 0.1% and this means if we are willing to dedicate the time and attention to a skill we want to learn, we already have the tools we need to succeed, it's about having the confidence to push ourselves up to that next level. Chiggs showed me what it takes to get better. I have never been a naturally artistic person, but I knew that with deliberate practice I could develop my skills and work towards providing the beautiful work that I saw him doing.

# Eustress

Stress gets a really bad rap. Stress is our natural response to a threat, shunting us into fight, flight or freeze mode, limiting our ability for rational thought as we prepare to take on, or off from, the immediate danger. As if acute stress isn't bad enough, chronic stress can cause long-lasting damage to our physical and mental wellbeing. When we're stressed, we can react angrily and with little provocation, we can flee at the first sign of trouble or procrastinate because we simply can't process any more meaningful information. Stress, however, is an also essential ingredient in our development.

Stress is our body's response to being pushed that little bit beyond where it is comfortable and it's the only way to improve. Eustress is the name given to the positive kind of stress that we encounter when we take on a physical or mental challenge that is just the right amount beyond our current skill level. When we exercise, we stress our bodies, creating micro-tears in our muscles leading to fatigue. In response, the body rebuilds our muscles stronger so the next time we come under the same stress we are better equipped to deal with it. Our brains work in a similar way, whether it's fatigue from complex decision-making or developing fine motor skills, our brains create more efficient neural pathways that help us improve our performance next time. Growth happens when we put ourselves through short and regular states of eustress.

"A smooth sea never made a skilled sailor."
**Franklin D. Roosevelt**

There's a fine balance between stress and eustress, but often what tips the balance is how we view the stress we're facing. When we're struggling to gain access into a fourth root canal in an upper molar it can be stressful, or we can view it as eustress, an opportunity to push ourselves to do something a little bit outside our comfort zone. At home, when my son was waking the whole house up five times a night it was exhausting and infuriating but it was also an opportunity to master the art of patience. When we face challenges, it's an opportunity to learn. Eustress is our mind's way of telling us we're on the right track. The most effective eustress is that which we plan and undertake proactively.

# Planning

Our brains have two systems of thinking. System 1 thinking, or our chimp brain, is for rapid processing so we can react quickly to a stimulus. Left unchecked, it usually results in us deciding to fight, flight or freeze. It's not rational, it's about speed and survival. It makes the fastest possible links from neurones A to B to C to keep us safe. System 1 kicks in when we're in a heightened state of alert (stress) and our hormones don't care whether it's serpents or surgery that have caused it.

System 2 processing, on the other hand, is our brain's more considered approach, when different parts of the brain can talk to each other and deduce more rational solutions than the reflexive System 1. It's our human brain, the rational, balanced thinking that we're allowed to do when we're not in immediate danger.

When we're tired, stressed or working under pressure, the adrenaline starts pumping to keep us going and our brains tend to operate more in System 1. If we're going to deliberately put ourselves under stress by pushing ourselves out of our comfort zone, we must make sure all the important decisions are made with System 2 thinking beforehand. We do this by planning. A clear guide formulated well before a procedure allows us to make the major decisions in a relaxed state with System 2 thinking, so we're not relying on System 1 during the stress of the moment. A comprehensive plan means breaking down each aspect of the treatment, deciding the best way to do it and making contingencies where there are foreseeable deviations.

Planning is an invaluable tool whatever level of dentistry you are undertaking. I used to make a plan for everything, right down to a small occlusal composite in my early days, and to this day, I still write a plan out for every implant surgery I undertake. My plan helps me relax during the procedure and it lets the rest of the team know what to expect on the day. The more relaxed we all are, the better we're going to work and communicate.

It's not possible to plan for every eventuality, but I find conducting what psychologist Gary Klein calls a pre-mortem is a valuable tool to identify where things may go wrong before they happen. Picture yourself at the end of a procedure, let's say a large filling on a molar. It's not gone well, there's a gap between the adjacent tooth and your restoration and you know you could have done better, so why has this happened? Maybe it was deeper than you expected, perhaps the filling on the tooth next door wasn't conducive to creating a good contact point, the gums were bleeding, the matrix band didn't fit, or a cusp broke off during treatment making the rebuild much harder.

With practice, none of these issues are insurmountable but they can be difficult when we're managing them for the first time, or if we're tired or stressed and our decision-making ability is reduced. If we can have the foresight to recognise these risks in our pre-mortem, we can plan in contingencies. We can make rational decisions when we're in a relaxed state of mind with our System 2 thinking and chances are, we're going to make much better choices about how to manage them than we would in the heat of the moment.

# Flow

Having a plan also allows me to get into the zone during a procedure, to really focus and work at my best. This is what Mihaly Csikszentmihalyi calls flow. Flow is a state of mind when we are completely immersed in a task that is just the right level of difficulty, fractionally beyond anything we've done before. When we reach a state of flow, we lose track of time, we have no other cares in the world aside from the singular skill that we are focusing on in that very moment. Finding a job or activity that allows you to regularly reach a state of flow gives us a very high level of satisfaction as well as promoting our personal development.

Reaching a state of flow gives me the sort of buzz that people jump from planes to get. I find flow when I place a dental implant and when I get into that zone, I know I'm performing at my best. Being in a state of flow means being completely immersed in the task at hand, free from distractions or other worries. It can feel like an escape, a freedom to give myself 100% to just one thing for a short period. In order to do this, when undertaking a complex procedure, the whole team needs to be involved. The whole team must understand that when we're getting in the zone, we can't be chatting about the weather, or have someone asking if we want a cup of tea. We need to minimise distractions so we can focus on the task at hand, but also that we need our team to check on the patient and keep an eye on the time, as we lose ourselves in the moment.

We don't have to be treating a patient to reach flow, we can achieve the same state with deliberate practice. I find this when I play piano, dedicating time to concentrate on one single activity with absolute focus allows me to reach flow. Deliberate practice is more than simply repeating the same process over and over, it's a constant cycle of planning, implementation and reflection that requires focus and an ability to keep pushing yourself to make things a little bit harder as soon as your actions begin to become mindless. Deliberate practice is hard, it takes sustained effort and a willingness to keep challenging ourselves. The sweet spot where our practice allows us to reach flow and puts us in a state of eustress is what leads to growth, but only with one more vital ingredient.

# Rest

Effective rest allows our brains to process new information from our deliberate practice. When I was learning to play Bohemian Rhapsody on piano, I found sections of the song were pushing my ability beyond anything I'd played before. The descending demisemiquavers of Brian May's guitar solo just prior to the operatic section of the song blew my mind, how was I ever going to be able to move my fingers that quickly. It felt pointless to even try.

When learning a new skill, we have to allow our brains to focus fully on the singular task at hand. We have to tell our brains that this task is important and it requires our full attention. By stripping the Bohemian Rhapsody solo back to its basic elements and focusing solely on playing the right hand at a speed I could manage, I was able to play it, even if it did sound like the version I used to hear when the batteries were going flat in my Walkman. I spent an hour practising the same four bars of music over and over again, but to my dismay, I was getting worse, not better. Each time I tried a bit harder to hit all the right notes and each time I'd make more mistakes. In a fit of frustration, I closed the lid of the piano.

A very strange thing happened the next day when I sat down to play again. On my first attempt at playing the same four bars of music, I played it better than I had managed at any point the day before. This blew my mind, how was it that I could play the same piece over and over again and not get any better, but the next day, I would be able to do it? The secret was in the rest. Sleep allowed my brain to upgrade its synaptic connections and by laying down new myelin it increased the efficiency of neural transmission so the next time I sat at my piano, my brain was more efficient at telling my fingers where to go. The repetition of the exercise told my brain that this was an important skill to learn and so when I gave it the opportunity to strengthen, it did so.

"Stress + Rest = Growth"
**Brad Stulberg**

Sleep is when our non-vital functions can switch off and our bodies can focus on restoring our strength, replenishing our immune system, healing and equilibrating. If you were in Professor Matthew Walker's study 'Practice with sleep makes perfect', you would have had your motor skills tested in the morning, again in the evening and once more after a full night's sleep. Your improvement would probably follow a predictable path, a rapid increase in skill after the first few attempts, followed by only slight improvements for the rest of the day. After a full night's sleep, you would show, on average, a sudden 20% improvement on the previous day's scores.

As if this wasn't testament enough to the power of sleep, the comparison group, first tested in the evening then the following morning and then again in the afternoon showed a similar pattern of big improvements after sleep and little improvement later in the day, despite being more practised. There was also a correlation in the study between participants getting good quality deep sleep with higher levels of improvement the following day.

Sleep is undeniably a key ingredient in the formula for growth. Not only do we perform worse if we haven't had enough sleep the night before, but we also don't learn effectively if we don't rest. If we fail to let our minds and bodies rest, we fail to give them the opportunity to strengthen regardless of how much eustress we put ourselves through.

# Coda

| Three steps to mastery |
|---|
| 1. Plan - A comprehensive plan including what might go wrong will minimise stress in the moment, lead to the best possible outcomes and maximise your learning. |
| 2. Eustress - Seek out activities that let you find a state of flow. These will be just challenging enough to push you slightly out of your comfort zone. |
| 3. Rest - Practice only makes perfect when we give our mind and body a chance to rebuild stronger. |

In order to consistently perform at our best, we need to maintain growth throughout our careers and this growth will only happen when we give ourselves direction and push ourselves out of our comfort zones, just enough to create eustress. We need to have confidence in our own ability and maintain a positive frame of mind that will give us strength in our convictions to keep going when times become challenging. Creating eustress in our lives and balancing this with appropriate rest is what will lead to growth.

The best time to stop doing something is when it becomes easy. When we feel completely comfortable carrying out a certain procedure, we've stopped learning. That's not to say we should stop providing that service for our patients, but we must realise that doing so is not going to help us provide better care in the future. It's easy to sit back and do only what we feel comfortable doing, and there are times when other stresses in our life might necessitate a relaxation from the relentless pursuit of improvement but, stopping our journey for too long will lead to stagnation and boredom. There is never an ideal time to step out of our comfort zone but to keep growing, we need to continually seek out new challenges, and attack them in a controlled way, with a clear plan, and a positive mindset.

There are many small things we can do to foster positivity, from focusing on our purpose to reframing our challenges as opportunities to grow. Life cannot always be lived in the positive though. There are times when it feels like self-improvement is impossible and the toxic positivity of someone telling you to reframe your negativity redoubles your pain. If we try to ignore our emotions, we put ourselves under even greater pressure. When we try to maintain an impeccable facade, we isolate ourselves from the people who may be able to support us. We can't always be positive, it's ok not to be ok.

# 7
# Bulletproof, I Wish I Was
## Radiohead

### *How to begin to understand mental health*

"Depression, seasonal and otherwise, turns all this upside
down: the past is a guilty place, the future a hanging
threat, the present a humiliation. Stop it, you want to
shout. Just stop it. Let me be."
**Horatio Clare - The Light in the Dark**

*I'm down at the moment. It happens every couple of months,
my mood dips, I feel hollow, vulnerable, irascible. I want to
lock myself away in a dark room and not talk to anyone,
not see anyone and maybe just cry for a bit. This shroud is
fogging my vision, my hearing, my taste, my appetite, my
voice, my life. I'm a ship at sea in the depth of a fantastic*

*storm, thunder crashing around me, the whole earth moving underneath my heavy bow and all I can do is lower the sails and pray it passes soon. The thought of sailing on to the next destination is impossible. I've reached the impasse and I have to wait until the clouds clear and I can resume my journey on calmer seas, hopefully without too much damage to myself or those around me. I'm generally energetic, positive and driven, I try to inspire those around me with passion and enthusiasm but right now that seems utterly preposterous. I can't even keep myself happy.*

The passage above is a diary entry from the summer of 2020 during a particularly low period. I chastise myself because I have no right to feel like this. I have a perfect life, this isn't meant as a boast but a statement of contentment with having a good job and a loving family. This subjugating spiral of sadness continues until I have lost all notions of self-worth. I tell myself that there are people far worse off than me, and I can't even cope with my cushy life, but knowing that some people have it worse doesn't help.

"Of course, there's always someone worse off than you. But imagine you're in a doctor's surgery with a broken arm. The person next to you has two broken arms, the person next to him has two broken arms and a broken leg. This is all very well, but the point is that you have a broken arm and it hurts."
**Robert Webb - How Not To Be a Boy**

Having a good life and a great mindset doesn't

immunise you against depression, just as they don't immunise you against a car crash or cancer. You wouldn't tell a friend, lying on the floor with a broken leg to pick themselves up, shake it off and come for a drink, and if you'd broken your leg, you wouldn't be afraid to tell your friend that you can't make it to your weekly game of badminton. Yet when it comes to mental illness, which can be incapacitating beyond most physical ailments, we still fall victim to these differing standards. The phrase 'it's ok to talk' still seems to be echoing in an empty room.

The stigma feels greater for healthcare professionals, we're the carers, the ones who look after others. As a professional, I believed that I should be unflinching in the face of adversity, with an unwavering constitution, never showing any signs of weakness or imperfection, no signs of being, well, human.

In 2019 the British Dental Journal published a study stating that almost half of all dentists say that the stress of their job is exceeding their ability to cope, and this was before the COVID pandemic hit. More than one in six dentists have seriously considered committing suicide at some point in their lives, with more than half of these dentists having thought about it in the last year. These startling figures say two clear things to me, firstly, if you're struggling, you are not alone, dentistry can be a very stressful job and you don't have to suffer in silence. Secondly, we must make sure we're looking after our own mental wellbeing if we want to be at our best for those around us.

*It appears to be that time again. I find myself plunged into the depths which seem so far away most of the time. I don't know how long I'll be here, the unpredictability is possibly the most difficult thing to comprehend, but I do know it's not permanent. I long for further understanding, some sort of logic behind it, but it all feels completely irrational. This isn't me, this gloom, this muffled cacophony inside my own Bell Jar, I can't reach out beyond the cold thick glass and the world outside seems a distant faraway land where everyone else is enjoying the sights, the sounds the smells that are all just shades of grey to me.*

Through keeping a diary, I noticed that these feelings were catching up with me every couple of months and they usually followed a period of high stress. It took me 33 years to begin to see this pattern. I'd be down for a few days, and then by the end of the week, I'd be energised and ready to take on the world again. I know now there is light at the end of the tunnel when I'm in that place and what's more, I usually bounce back higher than I was before. I'm stronger for having overcome my demons. I'm lucky that my suffering is limited to a few days every couple of months and when it hits, it's not nearly as bad as what many people go through.

I know my mental health has never been better than since I've taken the time to appreciate my own mental wellbeing. Whilst I still experience highs and lows, as everyone does, they don't inhibit me from living a full life and I've reached a point of acceptance of these fluctuations. There is a Buddhist philosophy about trying to control our emotions that changed the way I view my mental wellbeing.

Picture yourself standing on a beach, your emotions are the ocean's waves lapping at your feet, some of them good, some of them bad, some of them gentle, some so forceful they knock you off your feet and almost pull you out to sea. Trying to control our emotions is tantamount to trying to stop the good waves from breaking apart and trying to stop the bad waves from hitting the shore. We can become stressed if we try to prolong the good waves and we can fear the moment when they leave, just as we may want to avoid the bad waves altogether. As much as we may want to, we cannot possess complete control over our emotions just as we cannot change the tide. Once we learn to accept that these waves are coming and going, we can learn how to live with them. By accepting the eddies of emotions, we can enjoy the moments of pleasure and we can begin to ride the waves of discontent rather than being consumed by them.

Increasing the awareness of mental wellbeing, including making the available support known across the profession, is imperative in helping to prevent people from taking the most devastatingly irreversible of steps. I hope that this chapter gives you the strength to reflect on your mental wellbeing and maybe have a conversation with someone close to you no matter how mild or severe you perceive your own fluctuations in mood. People who suffer from low moods, depression or any form of mental ill-health can be very adept at hiding it, often they've had a lifetime of practice in doing so. By opening up the channels of conversation, we may just give somebody the opportunity to talk rather than bottle up, and that may make all the difference.

When I first shared my experience of a period of low mood, I received a lot of love and support from close family members and good friends who had no idea I had such episodes. A lot of people realised in that moment that you just don't know how someone is feeling, no matter how close they are. I'd managed to keep what felt like my dirty little secret, hidden from the people who cared about me the most. I thought I was insulating myself from the pain of exposure when really, I was isolating myself to suffer alone. What I found was that the people that matter didn't try to 'fix' me, they didn't offer advice, they just listened and were there for me. The shame I had felt about people finding out vanished the moment I opened up.

Being married to a psychotherapist has empowered me to be open about my mental wellbeing. It's through talking to Marisa that I've been able to identify some triggers and take steps to improve my mental wellbeing, so I can be a better husband, father, friend, and a better dentist. So much of what is written throughout these pages has been influenced by Marisa but the following sections titled In The Mind are written by her. Marisa gives her professional perspective on some of my experiences and insights into areas of mental health that I'm less familiar with. I've never met anyone like Marisa who can understand people on a level deeper than I knew existed and I know you'll find her contributions fascinating and helpful, whether it's for you or someone else.

## In The Mind

It is important to apply caution when using the term depression as there is of course a broad spectrum, with episodes of low mood at one end and clinical depression at the other. Clinical depression is more persistent and can have a devastating impact on daily functioning. Trying to draw comparisons between degrees of mental wellbeing across the spectrum is not helpful as everyone experiences these emotions differently, just as we all experience the common cold differently, and there is a whole host of external circumstances and factors at work. Furthermore, whether we find labels such as 'depression' useful or not, is an entirely individual choice, each person and situation is unique.

The qualities that make a great dentist, such as attention to detail, can easily become perfectionism which is detrimental to mental health. Dentists and other healthcare professionals have the desire to help people and fix things which, alongside the duty of care to patients, can become a heavy responsibility to carry. This is especially true in unfortunate situations where things cannot be fixed or when things go wrong. Working as a dentist requires high levels of concentration for several hours with very little time between patients for breaks. There is also the pressure of knowing a mistake could have negative implications for a patient's health. This creates an intense environment that is not helped when the very people you're trying to help, as it is generally perceived, don't like you. All this before we even consider the damaging effects that a persistent anxiety about complaints or litigation can cause.

Dentistry can also be an isolated role, working from one surgery with little opportunity for socialising or garnering support from colleagues, which is not an ideal foundation for building good mental wellbeing. Because of this, when problems do arise, the lack of support can be catastrophic. I can understand why many dentists find it hard to admit they're struggling, under the guise of maintaining the standards of being a professional on top of the general stigma that still exists about discussing mental health difficulties. I think that there's then an additional layer of guilt that prevents dentists from validating their own experiences as they work in, broadly speaking, a well-paid profession that they have trained for many years to achieve.

"Comparison is the thief of joy."
**Theodore Roosevelt**

We compare our internal thoughts and feelings to other people's external behaviour, this is especially true with social media, yet we are expected to only show socially acceptable behaviours and emotions. It's no wonder everyone else seems ok, while inside, we are far from it and we can easily conclude that it must be just us that feels like this. We can conclude that there must be something deficient within us when in fact, in my experience as a counsellor, the thing that is fundamentally wrong is usually something we have encountered that shapes our emotions; negative environments, relationships or experiences.

The focus should not be on what is 'wrong' with an individual, but on what has happened to them and what support they need to move forward and fulfil their potential. Erratic emotions are often perfectly normal responses to living in an abnormal world. This is a compassionate, humanistic stance that does not medicalise what it is to be human.

## Anxiety

Anxiety can take many forms, I'm fortunate that anxiety, as Marisa would use the term, is not something that I have had to battle with. My insights here therefore may seem trivial to some, however, I hope they add value to anyone who can relate to them.

Whilst I'm not generally affected by long-term anxiety, I do get pre-performance anxiety before a big procedure or public speaking. This anxiety kicks my brain and body into fight or flight mode so I can prepare to take action. This isn't a bad thing, it's exactly what I need to perform at my best, but it's exhausting. When the effects of the adrenaline stop, I need a lie down in a dark room to regroup before I'm ready to go again.

I see this when mentoring implant students. They're anxious before an implant procedure because they're stepping out of their comfort zone. Once the implant fixture is in, they relax and the adrenaline stops, just as they need to concentrate and use their usually well-honed fine motor skills for suturing. Placing a simple suture becomes the most difficult part of the procedure because they're exhausted, the adrenaline that kept them going has gone and they're running on empty.

If this brief rollercoaster is how pre-performance anxiety affects us, can you imagine what it must be like to be on the ride all day, every day? Anxiety that is ever present, burning up our resources can put us in a chronic state of stress. The relentless bombardment of stress hormones can leave us feeling permanently on the edge. We become trapped in fight or flight which turns off the rational parts of our brains that would normally help us find a way out of the situation. This anxiety may not have a readily identifiable source, but it can be worrying about future events that may never happen; a patient complaint, an altercation with a colleague, or worrying someone we care about may become ill.

In my first few weeks out in the real world of dentistry, I remember the trepidation when I spotted a molar root canal treatment in the diary in a week's time, the first one I'd done outside of dental school. I revised, planned and prepared but despite all this, I still harboured an anxiety that lasted until the appointment. I spent every waking moment fretting about what could go wrong. If we're not careful, we can spend so much energy worrying about what could go wrong, we fail to plan to do it right. To put it another way, by worrying so much about the outcome, we lose sight of the process. On top of this, my anxiety caused me to lose sleep, so I wasn't feeling at my best for the procedure, nor for anything else in the preceding days.

I notice the same feeling starting on occasions to this day, though I can identify and process these emotions better now. Once I've done my planning, I know the best thing I can do to prepare is to forget about it, rest, and approach the day with a refreshed mind. It's not a switch that can be turned off and on, but by identifying the cause and understanding that the long buildup of anxiety doesn't help, I've been able to compartmentalise my emotions and this allows me to prepare far better than weeks of worrying would.

In The Mind

Anxiety is a future-based fear leading to hyperarousal due to the activation of the fight or flight response. This can be due to external factors, such as perceived danger, or internal factors, a conflict within yourself such as when your self-concept and core values are at odds with your life experiences or relationships. It can affect people in many ways, there may be an inability to function, an avoidance of anxiety-provoking situations, sleep disturbances, physical symptoms, digestive disturbances, muscle pain, bruxism, or an inability to maintain relationships to list a few. The overthinking that often accompanies anxiety can overwhelm the brain leading to a paralysing level of fear, phobias, social anxiety and panic attacks.

We all experience anxiety in response to specific situations like an exam or job interview, this is a natural and often useful response which subsides once the event has finished. It is only problematic when it is persistent and impacts our ability to function normally in daily life. It may be that anxieties triggered by single events need addressing through therapy, but anxiety can also be an accumulation of smaller things or a response to prolonged exposure to a toxic environment.

As if the sensation of feeling anxious isn't bad enough, we often then use a significant amount of our body's resources in trying to ignore or fight these feelings. Even if we can do this successfully, simply dealing with the symptoms of anxiety is like taking painkillers for a toothache, it may help numb the pain for a while, but there's still a bad tooth in your mouth that needs sorting. Identifying the anxiety is the first step, often it's by noticing the physical signs that allow us to recognise the underlying cause.

Let's replace the word anxiety with allergy for a moment. You may have noticed that you get an allergic reaction sometimes, the symptoms are often similar but they're not always identical. Initially, you don't know what you're allergic to, you may not even realise it's an allergy, and you expend a great amount of energy into fighting the reaction. In time, however, you can spot patterns, identify certain triggers, or see the warning signs when the symptoms are less severe. Reframing a mental issue with a physical one isn't always helpful, but in this instance, the allergy analogy can give you the self-awareness that allows you some psychological distance from the symptoms. You can start to use your energy to identify the source of the problem instead of fighting with the reaction.

We can't always avoid our 'allergens' but some of our most effective 'antihistamines' for anxiety are self-care, mindfulness and talking. Using these tools, we can keep the frequency and intensity of our reactions lower and our recovery is much quicker.

Sometimes, we can't identify the cause of our anxiety, it may be buried deeper within us, caused by something in our past, or perhaps we can identify it but are unable to process the emotions on our own to be able to function normally. It's at these times that reaching out for support is most important, whether it's to a friend, or by seeking further support. Anxiety can be extraordinarily debilitating, but it is not something that you need to put up with. You can do something about it.

## Intrusive Thoughts

*I've been feeling a bit flat, tired from a busy period of work, probably teetering towards burnout. Today, I've been lecturing in Manchester, something I love doing but takes a lot of preparation and a lot of energy, so by the end of the day I was exhausted. On my way home, leaving the motorway at 70mph, on the slip road, the thought went through my mind that I could just choose not to brake as I careered towards the roundabout. I could just let whatever happens, happen. It was a moment of apathy for everything, an unwanted, unpleasant fleeting thought of just letting go.*

*The moment passed, my car slowed and my mind raced. What the heck was that? What does it mean? I don't feel depressed. I'm not suicidal. Is my subconscious trying to hijack me? Is this the start of a slippery slope that will one day defeat me?*

I only found out about intrusive thoughts a couple of years ago when I first had one and it scared the life out of me. I worried that this was a big step in the wrong direction with my mental health. The most important thing I did when this happened was to talk to someone, as usual for me, this was Marisa.

<u>In The Mind</u>

Intrusive thoughts are common, most people get them and they're not a sign that you're on a slippery slope to suicide. Even suicidal ideations aren't uncommon, they aren't anything more than thoughts. You are not your thoughts and it's ok to have them. It's worth speaking about your intrusive thoughts to someone, a friend, a relative or a counsellor but I hope it does offer some reassurance that, in most instances, they are completely normal. They're only a problem if they're constantly intruding on your life, causing constant distress, or if they become conscious ideations, rather than unwanted intrusions. At this point, it's time to seek professional help. At the most severe end of the scale, some people feel compelled to comply with intrusive thoughts, for example, those with Obsessive Compulsive Disorder.

There is understandably a lot of fear surrounding suicide, so much so, people often try to avoid talking about it, but the reality is that by openly having a conversation about suicide, we reduce the chances of someone acting on their thoughts. We need to allow the space, time and opportunity for those thoughts to be talked through. This breaks the isolation for that individual and enables them to receive support. If you can take away only one thing from any of my contributions in this book, let it be to be brave in your conversations with others where suicide might just be beneath the surface. If you are having these thoughts, be brave in opening up to someone and if someone raises the courage to talk to you, be brave enough to listen to them without judgement.

# Coda

| Three steps to mastery |
| --- |
| 1. It's ok not to be ok. You don't need to have a reason, you don't need to judge yourself or compare your situation to anyone else. |
| 2. Understand your experiences are unique. The ones I've shared may be nothing like your own and it's understanding that everyone experiences a range of emotions that allows us to be human. |
| 3. Don't expect to find a quick fix or a cure that will magically make all your emotions disappear, though there are many ways we can strengthen our mental wellbeing. |

There once lived a very skilled cobbler in a large village. As the only cobbler for miles, everyone went to him to repair their shoes and this kept him so busy that he didn't have time to repair his own boots. This wasn't a problem at first, but over time, his boots began to wear and fall apart. His feet got blisters and he started to limp while the rest of the village walked around happily. Even when his friends started to worry, he would reassure them that everything was fine and he kept fixing everyone else's shoes but neglecting his own.

After a few years, the cobbler was so debilitated, he could hardly walk and was no longer able to work properly. He wasn't able to fix the shoes of even those closest to him and as a result, the entire town started to limp in pain. By neglecting his own needs, he was ultimately unable to help the people who needed him.

If we can't take the time to care for ourselves, pretty soon, we'll find we can't care for anyone else. We must prioritise our own mental wellbeing to allow for personal development and enable us to continue to help the people around us. The experiences I've shared in this chapter are my own, some people may have experienced something similar, and others will have had completely different experiences.

The solutions are equally diverse, if they can even be called solutions. We can optimise our physical health with regular exercise and a balanced diet and this reduces the likelihood of us falling ill, though it will never protect us from all maladies. Exercise and diet can also help our mental wellbeing, but of course, professional athletes and nutritionists still suffer from physical and mental health conditions. There is no one size fits all solution, nor a vaccine that can immunise us against negative emotions but there are many good habits we can build to strengthen our mental wellbeing.

# 8

# Feeling Good
## Nina Simone

### *How to strengthen your mental wellbeing*

"Until you make the unconscious conscious, it will direct
your life and you will call it Fate."
**Carl Jung**

For a long time, I tried to fight the waves of my
emotions, telling myself I didn't have a problem, perhaps
for fear of labelling myself. I've never been diagnosed
with a mental health condition or felt the need to seek
further help beyond talking to Marisa and my close
friends, but what I failed to see is that the lack of
attention I gave to my mental wellbeing meant that when
my mood did fluctuate, it was unsettling for everyone
around me.

A manic phase would stress everyone around me as they were unable to keep up with my constant need to do more more more and I would end up burning out. My mood and energy levels would dip, I would become either irascible or completely apathetic. I could keep it together and be professional when I was with a patient but then I might lash out at a friend. I would fail to look after myself and I'd certainly be unable to support the people around me.

I realised that this was not a sustainable way of living. I needed to change something if I was to be able to be the kind of father, husband, friend, and dentist I wanted to be. There were two things I did that improved my mental wellbeing and my life. The first was increasing my self-awareness, and the second was talking more openly about mental health.

## Self-Awareness

Keeping a daily journal was the first step in improving my self-awareness. As my habit developed, I explored my thoughts and feelings more and the further I dove introspectively, the greater I came to appreciate the ebbs and flows of my mood.

My journal, which I still call my one line a day, though it's considerably more than that now, is purely for me. Nobody else will ever read it and this allows me to write uncensored, so I can process my thoughts without fear of being judged. I will not be held to account for what I've written and so my emotions, no matter how irrational, can be vented, giving me clarity and perspective. Once they're written down, I don't have to carry them with me any longer, if I don't need or want to.

Through keeping a journal, I've been able to see myself more clearly. I can see the patterns of mania followed by burnout. I can see that when I was manic, I was too focused on work, I neglected my family and when I was down, I was unable to do anything. Armed with this knowledge, I knew it was time for me to take action to improve my mental wellbeing. I wasn't searching for a permanent cure, but I wanted to take ownership of my mental health and ride the waves of my emotions instead of fighting them.

A final addition to my daily journal was to take a moment to write down one thing every day that I'm grateful for, a practice that research shows has a positive impact on our mental wellbeing. Appreciating the big and the small things in life helps put everything into perspective. Even when we find ourselves in highly stressful periods, we can take solace in the small joys.

In The Mind

You can't pour from an empty cup. Many of my clients put themselves near the bottom of their own priority list for too long. If we fail to love ourselves, look after our body and mind, manage our stress levels and seek out support when we need it, we are setting ourselves up to fail. We don't deliberately neglect ourselves, we just don't take the time to reflect on our own emotions and needs, so we lack an awareness of our wellbeing. It's easier to plough forward, focusing on everyone else than to look inside ourselves. We keep planning for the future without seeing that the destination is not the heaven that we envisaged, and we put ourselves through hell to get there.

Three steps to self-awareness

1. Slow down. You do not need to fill every spare second with the next task or a phone screen.
2. Do one thing at a time. I get it, there's always more to do, but if you're going to do something, do it well and give that one thing your full attention.
3. Take mindfulness breaks. Set specific points in your day to take stock of how you are feeling physically and mentally. Is your breathing calm and your mind clear? Or is your body tense and your mind busy? You might want to write down what you notice down, journalling your thoughts has a huge therapeutic benefit, helps you identify patterns and triggers for anxiety and improves your self-awareness.

My clients often tell me how empowering it feels to increase their self-awareness, as they now have the choice of continuing as they were or making changes. Change is not compulsory and it's not always necessary, sometimes greater levels of understanding and awareness are all that are needed to improve mental wellbeing and opens the door to further areas of personal development.

# Mindfulness

I have been guilty of charging through life, failing to take notice of the world around me or inside me. Mindfulness is a humbling experience that allows me to turn off autopilot and take a moment to appreciate the awesomeness of the world around me and how I'm just a very small part of something much, much greater.

Practising mindfulness has allowed me to savour the little moments in life, like a crisp intake of Yorkshire air in winter, the first mouthful of a lovingly prepared meal or the bitterness of Citra and Mosaic hops in my dry hopped IPA on a Friday evening. Beyond the physical sensations, mindfulness empowers me to identify and accept my emotions in a moment of pain, pleasure, rage, rapture, frustration or freedom. Everything I know about mindfulness, I have learned from Marisa.

In The Mind

To be mindful is to focus our attention on each moment with greater awareness of what we are doing, thinking and feeling, emotionally and physically. It is to take notice without judging our feelings or trying to change them. It's hard to be anxious if you are truly mindful. If anxiety is based in the future, depression is often focused on the past, and mindfulness is about keeping ourselves in the present moment. Mindfulness is rooted in ancient Buddhism and it's a powerful tool that has never been more relevant to our modern Western culture. It's less about learning something new and more about unlearning a lifetime of holding on to external pressures.

Our lives are becoming overwhelming, with ever-greater demands on our time and attention. Most of us always have a smartphone within touching distance with countless group chats, the infinite scroll of social media and the feeling that we need to be accessible 24 hours a day. We are told from a young age that we need to do more, multitask, tick things off lists, hit goals, keep an eye on the time, do more and do it faster. The insurmountable expectations of being ever-present, ever-doing, prevent us from switching off, affecting both our physical and mental health. Sometimes the simplest solution such as a digital detox, even just a short-term one, is an opportunity to simplify our living and reduce competing demands.

How many times have you reached somewhere, home or work, and realised you had not consciously thought about your route? This is an example of acting on autopilot, you are disconnected from the moment, your surroundings and what you are actually doing. By increasing our awareness of the present moment, we can experience a renewed appreciation for our environment and the people around us that we may have been taking for granted. Have you ever noticed that preschool children never rush? They all have mindfulness nailed. Children are our best mindfulness teachers; they are fully present in each moment and they don't judge themselves for what they're doing or how they're feeling.

By rediscovering our inner child, that innate curiosity with our surroundings, we can shake off the years of conditioning to *do,* and instead, we can start to *be.* Mindful living increases self-awareness, as we separate ourselves from our thoughts and notice patterns in our emotions. We can learn to identify our warning signs for stress and take steps to stop ourselves from reaching burnout and by recognising our thought patterns, we can make informed choices to avoid toxic thoughts.

Warning: Mindfulness is a powerful tool. When you start practising mindfulness you may become aware of difficult thoughts or feelings, you may initially feel more emotional discomfort and may want to seek additional support to work through the feelings you have become aware of.

Like any new skill, it does take practice but by starting small and allocating a regular window to be mindful, you can start a new habit that will stick and once you feel the well-being mindfulness can bring, you will reap the benefits every day for the rest of your life.

Three steps to mindfulness

1. Take notice during your everyday activities and focus on what effect each activity is having on each of your senses, one by one. How does the water feel as you wash your hands? Warm? Cold? Can you feel the bubbles on your skin? What does the soap smell like? Notice the sound of the running water and how it

cascades off your hands. Small intermissions in your day-to-day living like this are simple yet effective for interrupting your own autopilot.

2. Watch your thoughts. Like clouds passing by, they come and go. Notice the different sizes, shapes, colours and weights of your thoughts as they float past. Don't get hooked into judging the thought or yourself for having it, try not to think of solutions, just appreciate their presence. You may notice your mind wandering, especially when you first try this, either replaying past problems or pre-empting future problems, try to bring yourself back to refocus your attention to this present moment and how you feel right now.

3. Label your thoughts. You are not your thoughts. By developing an awareness of them and giving them a label, for example, 'this is the fear of failure thought again', you can create some distance between yourself and your thoughts and feelings.

These three simple steps are a gentle introduction to mindfulness that will bring some calm into your day allowing you to be less stressed and more grounded in the present moment. When you are living in the moment you will experience benefits to your wellbeing and happiness. Additionally, your greater capacity to connect with those around you will help your relationships inside and outside work. This is just the beginning, utilising mindfulness techniques is something you may wish to develop further, but these three steps will certainly help you be present in the moment and improve your self-awareness.

A further extension of mindfulness is meditation, which involves sitting or laying in silence whilst you become aware of your thoughts, breathing or any tension in your body. Again, it's normal to catch your mind wandering, acknowledge this without judgement and refocus your attention on your body. Taking as little as sixty seconds is enough to clear your mind and allow you to reconnect with both yourself and the present moment. Many physical and mental health benefits result from meditating, including increased clarity in your thinking, reduced stress levels and an increased capacity to withstand stressful situations when they do occur.

There are many apps and courses available that can help with mindfulness and meditation. The right yoga class is also a great way to get started. Yoga is not all about seeing who can contort themselves into the most bizarre position. Much of yoga is about self-awareness, mindfulness and having an understanding of your body.

## Talking

Nobody possesses a bulletproof mind, immune to the highs and lows of life, yet we can still find it difficult to admit to ourselves that we have periods of low mood, depression, anxiety or any mental health label. We all live on a spectrum of emotional states at any one point in time, everybody is on the same spectrum. If admitting it to ourselves is difficult, it can feel even more daunting to talk to somebody else. Being able to talk openly and listen without casting judgement is a display of great strength. When I started to open up about my lows, I felt a surge of confidence as I could show that, while this is a part of me, a part of being human, it does not define me and I am stronger for taking ownership of this aspect of my life instead of pretending it doesn't exist.

I first publicly 'came out' about my mental wellbeing in a blog post and I've been asked if I worry about what other people think about me. If any one of my friends, family or even patients has a problem with me admitting that I am human, then they're not the kind of people I need or want in my life. There have been a few people who've tried to 'fix me' by prescribing more exercise or a better diet, these comments are always from people who don't really know me. The biggest impact of sharing my feelings is that I've grown closer to every person that is important to me. I've had friends open up to me about their own difficulties and I've made new friends who've placed their confidence in me as someone who may just understand how they feel. I hope that by being open about my struggles, I give someone else the strength to open up and just maybe they'll feel as empowered and liberated as I have for doing so.

Being dentists, we want to help people. We diagnose and treat the problems we encounter, making us the fixers for other people's problems. This is great when it's teeth, a subject we've spent at least five years studying to treat, but when it's about mental health, we are woefully underqualified to help. This can lead us to either offer bad advice or avoid these difficult conversations altogether. If someone does feel that you are the person that they need to talk to, the solution is so simple that it is often overlooked. Just listen. When I'm in that place, having someone to talk to, to process my own emotions without fear of judgement, is often all I need. That said, I often don't need or want to talk at all in those moments, so this should never be forced upon someone. I don't need solutions or reassurance, just having someone willing to listen when I'm ready to talk is enough to empower me to start taking steps out of the darkness.

## In The Mind

Listen with empathy, regardless of your opinion, the person who is opening up to you is going through a hard time. Even with the best intentions, 'look on the bright side' type comments dismiss the validity of that person's feelings and can silence them from opening up again. It takes a great deal of courage and vulnerability to share emotions and experiences. Maybe you don't want to hear what they have to say, maybe you're too busy or feel you don't have the skills, this is ok too. You don't need to take on everyone's problems, but try not to disregard their emotions with toxic positivity which may make them feel worse. Acknowledge that what they've shared sounds difficult and either keep listening or help them find somewhere where they can get more support.

You can ask if there is anything you can do for them and it's ok to offer advice if it's been asked for. If it's a colleague, you may want to set some time aside to check in with each other a bit more regularly, a walk together on lunch or a phone call after work. Where possible, try to be considerate of what the other person may be going through and how the difficulties may affect their daily life. For instance, during a depressive episode, it can be harder to get started in the morning, so a patient who is struggling may prefer appointments later in the day. By contrast, an anxious patient may prefer your first appointment of the day to avoid their anxiety building throughout the day. You may also see patterns in your colleagues' behaviour, sometimes simply labelled as someone 'not a morning person', maybe they just need a little more space first thing. Difficult conversations may be better saved for later in the day with these people.

Talking about mental wellbeing still carries a stigma, perhaps one day this won't be the case, but for now, we know these conversations don't come naturally to most people, whether you're the person who is struggling or if you're the person they've reached out to. If nothing else, simply being there and listening with an understanding ear is often enough to allow someone to work through their thoughts and find their way to a better place.

# Coda

| Three steps to mastery |
|---|
| 1. Keep a personal journal to help you identify your emotions and recognise patterns in your mood. |
| 2. Try Marisa's three steps to self-awareness on page 126 and mindfulness on page 129 and notice how you feel after taking these mindful moments. |
| 3. Talk about mental wellbeing. The more we have these conversations, the more comfortable everyone will become with them. You never know when someone may just need someone to talk to. |

It has taken a long time for me to begin to come to terms with my mental wellbeing. There have been lows on my journey, but with each one I've learned a little more about myself and by improving my self-awareness, through talking and keeping a journal, I've started to understand my mind, my rhythms and my triggers a little better. The combination of writing and talking is enough to help me work through the difficult times I've faced. If you're supporting someone else, simply being present and listening is often enough to help.

There are times when we may need more support. Confidental is a charity that provides an ear for dentists, hygienists, therapists and students in crisis, or those who need to talk to someone. The profits from this book are going to support the fantastic work that they do. Find Confidental online or by calling 0333 987 5158.

Marisa Walker-Finch is a BACP accredited psychotherapist who supports her clients with anxiety, depression, loss, stress and traumatic life events amongst many other things. She also has a unique insight into the challenges we can face in dentistry. Distance is no longer a barrier to care as she sees most of her clients online. Find Marisa online or by calling 07538 798025.

There is no panacea for mental wellness, but there are many ways we can strengthen our mental wellbeing as we would our physical health and in doing so, we can continue our journey of growth. Resilience does not mean never getting knocked down, it is the ability to keep getting back up again. I know I will experience lows again throughout my life, but I feel now that whilst I can't control the tides of emotion, I don't have to fight them. The bad waves may lap upon the shore and I'm ready to ride them. I am stronger for being aware of my mental health and empowered to maintain the passion I have for dentistry.

When we love our work, we can start to blur the lines between work and play. I don't believe we should be working to live or living to work, but we require both sides to coexist to build a fulfilling career and life. We have to find a way to establish a stable work-life balance so we can live and love both to the fullest.

# 9

# Eight Days a Week

## The Beatles

### *How to establish the right work-life balance*

"The only route to psychological freedom is to let go of the fantasy of getting it all done and instead to focus on doing a few things that count."
**Oliver Burkeman**

It's cold outside, and grey, and wet, the kind of day when I could quite happily stay inside and watch a film, or two, or binge a series, or two. But, it's 7 am, and I've got a patient at 830. I love my job, but I love my family too and there's a moment when I look across the breakfast table at the little faces, smiling at me through a putrescent crust of snot and Weetabix, that's calling me to stay at home today. As I stand up to leave, my daughter starts wailing uncontrollably that she doesn't want me to go, generating more of the limitless supply of fresh snot that she's determined to smear all over my new Hugo Boss chinos.

Family may not always be glamorous but it's the most important part of my life. I want to be with the people I love as much as possible, but I also want to be the best dentist I can be, the best mentor, the best lecturer, blogger, writer, and the best friend. I need to earn a certain amount of money to keep putting food on the table, but I don't want to finish work on Friday so exhausted that I need the whole weekend to recover, just to go back to work again on Monday. I need to look after myself too, physically and mentally. I need exercise and I love playing piano, and guitar, and reading, and writing. There is an infinite amount of stuff to do and as Oliver Burkeman highlights so dramatically, I'm only going to live for Four Thousand Weeks. There's simply not enough time to fit everything in.

Burnout is an incapacitating overload of stimuli. It follows a period of intense stress that pushes us to a point where our brain is unable to function effectively. When I reach the point of burnout I descend into a period of apathy, where my mind ceases to function as it once did, I struggle to make even basic decisions, such as what to wear or eat. I harbour feelings of inadequacy; I convince myself that I am barely capable of doing even routine dentistry. I'm in no condition to try to step out of my comfort zone to improve. In this state of mind, I can't be at my best for my patients or my loved ones. Time away from work becomes all about recovery so I can go back to work again, consequently, the most important people in my life never get me at my best.

Four thousand weeks is the blink of an eye in cosmological terms and not nearly enough time for any one person to do everything. It is, however, an exceptionally long period if we consider that it's a miracle we're here in the first place. We have this precious gift of life and consciousness, and we have the opportunity to make the very best of it if we choose to apply ourselves. Every decision that we make is also a decision not to do any one of an infinite number of other things we could be doing with our time. By embracing this notion, we can ensure that the choices we make are the most important ones and once we've made the choice not to do everything else, we need to apply ourselves with purpose. But choosing to do only the most important things is only half the battle.

Elite sports teams don't maintain a high-intensity attack for a whole match, they plan and choose the most effective time to push hard and when to conserve energy. If we want to consistently perform at our best, we need to find a way of exerting our energy most effectively. This balance of high intensity and relaxation is different for everyone, and I want to share the way I found the best balance for me, so I could give the best version of me to the people who matter most.

# HUSTLE + hush

A couple of years ago I piggybacked on one of Marisa's webinars and discovered Tee Twyford, a psychosynthesis qualified leadership coach who introduced me to a concept that revolutionised the way I use my time and energy. One of Tee's signature workshops, the Energy Map, helped me find the optimal balance between high energy, high performance, or HUSTLE activities, and lower energy, rest and recharge, or hush. Using Tee's HUSTLE and hush concept I was able to identify my strengths when I'm performing at my best and my weaknesses when I'm depleted. Knowing this, I've been able to modify my work-life balance to allow me to consistently perform at my best when I need to.

Tee has very kindly allowed me to share this process with you here, so grab a pen and paper and invest a few minutes to give yourself a much deeper understanding of how to use your time with maximal impact.

First, make a list of ten words that describe you when you're at your best. These will be positive words like passionate, relaxed, confident, stoic or happy. Now make another list of words that represent how you feel right now. These may be positive or negative and include feelings like anxious, driven, exhausted, creative or angry. You are allowed to feel opposing emotions at any one point in time, you can feel stressed and relaxed if you've had a manic day but are currently sitting in your pyjamas reading this book.

The HUSTLE + hush Energy Map in figure 1 is split into quadrants, with high and low energy on the vertical axis, and positive and negative on the horizontal.

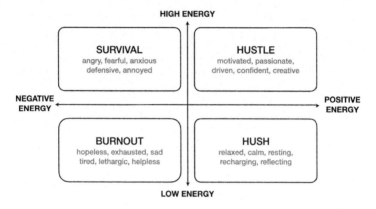

Figure 1. HUSTLE + hush Energy Map

The upper half is our high energy zone, all these are emotions that use a lot of our resources, anger, anxiety, passion, and confidence. Below is our low energy zone, containing things like apathy, hopelessness, calmness, and reflective. On the right side, we have our positive emotions and on the left our negative ones.

I want you to place the words you used to describe yourself at your best, on the energy map. They should all be on the right-hand side in the positive zone because they're you at your best, this is where we want to spend all of our time if we can. Note down the balance between HUSTLE, your high energy positive words in the top right of the map, and hush, your low energy positive words in the bottom right.

My HUSTLE:hush balance was 7:3, meaning that to perform at my peak, I need to reserve 30% of my time for doing low-intensity activities, to enable me to sustain my performance in high-intensity activities. If I am spending more time than this on high-intensity activities, I'm likely to fall towards burnout. A low-intensity activity isn't necessarily unproductive and it doesn't just mean sitting and reading a book, though it could be. Low-intensity activities are anything that doesn't require high amounts of energy, writing treatment plan letters, completing simple CPD, or even ironing or washing the dishes.

The left side of the map is made up of Survival and Burnout. Survival, in the top left corner of the map, is the use of high amounts of energy on negative emotions, anxiety, stress, and anger, all these things use up a lot of our resources without having a positive impact on our lives. Burnout, in the bottom left, comes when we have very little energy left and what little we have, we use in an unproductive way.

Now take a moment to place the words describing how you currently feel on the map. How do these words fit in compared to your best self? Do you have a similar split between high and low energy and how many of the words are falling on the negative side?

If you find your current balance isn't quite right, it's time to take action. When I did this, I found I had a balance of 7:3 high to low energy, but startlingly, the low energy feelings were on the left side, in the burnout zone.

When we spend too long hustling, without dedicating time to hush, we can find ourselves in survival mode and eventually burned out. I was constantly working at a high intensity, achieving a lot but then I'd suddenly crash and I'd have no explanation for it. Tee's Energy Map highlighted where I was going wrong. I hadn't been able to see that, to perform consistently at my best, I need to build in positive hush time, rather than trying to always hustle. I kept pushing and pushing myself and expected my brain and my body to keep up and when they inevitably failed, I became no use to anyone.

The key then is maintaining a balance by planning and using our time in harmony with our mind and body's capabilities. In Tee's words, to 'HUSTLE smarter and hush deeper'. By planning in hush time, we can use our low-energy time positively while also allowing us to perform at our best when we're hustling. I have been able to structure my time so that all my HUSTLE time, the time when I'm at my best, wasn't given exclusively to my patients, but also to my family and friends. In an always-on culture where we are trying to be all things, to all people, all of the time, embracing hush in my life permitted me to stop. It empowered me to take some time out of my busy schedule because I knew that I'd be stronger in the short and long term for doing so.

## CAPping Time

There was a time when I would be working five days on a full clinic, in addition to the time needed to plan cases, write letters to patients or colleagues and study for my master's. The inevitable result was less time with my family, a constant task list weighing on my mind during clinics, inefficiently planned treatment sessions and a perpetual level of stress about not having time to get everything done. Something had to give, I wasn't spending any time in the present moment, my work hours were lost to feelings of guilt about not being with my family, and my family time was spent fretting about work. I have found the most effective way of keeping myself in the moment is to implement clear boundaries on my time. In doing so, I can dedicate meaningful time to my family and work productively when I'm away from home. It is because I maintain discipline with my time that I have the freedom to enjoy it.

As dentists, we have three types of time available to us; clinical (C), admin (A) and personal (P).

## Clinical time

Clinical time is the time we spend with a dental chair at our disposal and a team around us to help care for patients. It is the most expensive time we have because it's our main source of income. The overheads on our clinical time are also huge and so it's important we don't waste it. This means making sure we do everything in our power to avoid having unplanned gaps in our diary and using the time with patients efficiently. A lot of our clinical time is spent hustling, using high amounts of energy in building relationships, making clinical decisions and focusing on providing a high level of care.

Admin time

Admin time is non-clinical time where we're not using a practice's resources and when often we don't directly derive an income. Scheduling admin time is an effective way to plan in some hush. It typically requires a lower amount of energy but that doesn't mean it can't be useful. Admin time is our opportunity to undertake CPD, to reflect on our learning, significant events, our purpose, and our direction and it's time to plan treatment sessions so we can use our clinical time most efficiently.

We can also plan more complex courses of treatment in a relaxed mindset, engaging our System 2 thinking, instead of making snap decisions during a busy clinic. We can use this time to complete other administrative tasks like writing letters, liaising with labs and colleagues or even writing articles or researching for publications. You may choose to use this time to shadow a mentor or explore another area of interest that you wouldn't ordinarily get a chance to explore.

Admin time is as valuable as you make it, but it does take practice to get good at using it. It helps to have a task list to work through and I'd strongly recommend that you plan what you hope to achieve during a session. Like all the best things in life, there is no immediate pay-off, but it will add considerable value to your life and work in the long term. Allocating dedicated admin time means that we can use our clinical time more efficiently and protect our personal time which can otherwise be overrun.

Personal time

If clinical time is the most expensive time, personal time is the most valuable. I guard it fiercely because it's my time with my family, my friends and time for my hobbies and exercise. What you choose to do in your personal time is entirely up to you, that's why it's personal time. However, without placing strong boundaries on our personal time, it can easily become overrun with a myriad of odds and ends that are left over from work.

If we fail to plan how we spend our time, we can find ourselves trying to shoehorn admin into our expensive clinical time or sacrifice personal time to catch up with work. CAPping our time liberates us to be completely present in each moment, knowing we have structured our lives as we want to live them. By maintaining discipline over how we use our time, we have the freedom to spend our personal time doing the things that are most important to us. However you choose to use your time, use it with purpose. Remember that every decision to do something is a decision not to do everything else.

# HUSTLE + hush and CAPping in Action

I needed to redress my HUSTLE + hush balance to a 7:3 ratio where my calmer time was planned in the hush zone, rather than burnout, in keeping with me at my best. I also applied my principle of CAPping time and the conclusion I came to was that I needed to reduce my clinical time. This would mean less high-intensity time on clinic, making more HUSTLE available for my personal time. It also meant planning in admin time for some work-related hush, which would allow me to coordinate my clinics and treatments better and not waste any of my clinical time on admin. In this way, I spend longer performing at my best

I reduced my clinical time by 20% and I estimated that I would have a 20% drop in income as a result. This was a sacrifice I was willing to make if it meant I'd have a better balance in my life with more time with my family and less time worrying about the number of things that weren't getting done. I'd rather live a 100% life on 80% of the money than an 80% life on 100% income. I do also acknowledge that I was fortunate to be in a position where I could accept a 20% reduction in income and this may not be the case for everyone.

To my amazement, at the end of the year, far from having a 20% reduction in income, I had actually earned more money. The 20% reduction in time spent sitting behind a dental chair had been dwarfed by a 50% increase in productivity of my clinical time. Not only this, but I felt happier, less fatigued, and I had the time to embrace some other opportunities that have resulted in further benefits that I would have never been able to enjoy had I been on clinic the whole time.

Mastering the perfect 60-second crown preparation is of no use if you start working on the wrong tooth. By giving ourselves time to plan appropriately, we can use our time more effectively and if we have the time to plan our care thoroughly, we will feel more confident in our ability to undertake more complex treatments and grow. I have been on a journey, at first I tried to work quickly, and I burnt out. Then I tried to work efficiently, I'd get more done but I'd still burn out. Now I feel like I'm working effectively. I'm using my time and energy in the best possible way to be able to give my best care to my patients and the best version of myself to my family.

# Priorities

With a system in place that allows us to consistently perform at our best, all we need to do now is decide what to do, particularly during our admin time. We're used to spending time caring for patients, working to a schedule that's already laid out for us. Our admin time is free from these constraints, but this often leads us to procrastinate or we can feel overwhelmed by trying to do too many things at once. Everyone's priorities are different and so what you choose to do with your time may be completely different to mine. When there are an infinite number of things we can do with our time, we need to use a simple system that will maximise our productivity, to ensure we're spending our time on the things that are most important to us.

<u>Three steps to prioritisation</u>

1. Split your tasks into three lists, headed A, B and C, in order of priority, with the A's being the most important tasks that will best help you work towards your purpose. The simple process of doing this in

itself gives you time to reflect, providing clarity and direction.

2. Throw the C list in the bin. There are so many things that you can do with your time that if it's already so far down as to be in the C category, it's clearly not a priority. The sooner you can remove these distractions, the better.

3. Do the A's first.

I've tried all manner of systems to find what works for me, from Eisenhower matrices to productivity apps that give me a dopamine-laden badge for ticking five jobs off in one day. I found the simplicity of one single list to be king. One list to rule them all. One list with only the most important things that will help me fulfil my purpose. The most important tasks are usually the ones that don't offer an immediate pay-off but are an investment that helps me develop my process.

# Coda

| Three steps to mastery |
| :--- |
| 1. Do Tee's HUSTLE + hush exercise. Figure out what balance allows you to consistently perform at your best. |
| 2. CAP your time. Schedule your admin time and boundary your personal time so you can give the best of you to the people who matter most. |
| 3. Set your priorities for your admin time using the three steps on page 148 to make sure the things you do are meaningful and align with your purpose. |

I don't want to retire when I'm 50, 60 or even 70. I want to build a long, happy and fulfilling career that allows me to keep working, to keep helping people, and to keep realising my purpose, long after everyone else's passion has burned up. I also don't want to work so hard now, saving for an early retirement, that I don't enjoy these years of my life, with a young family and an able body.

To enable me to have this long, passionate career, I need to maintain a balance in my life and I found the right balance for me using Tee Twyford's HUSTLE + hush exercise. To reach the right balance, I reduced my clinical time and planned regular admin time. Not only has this made my clinical time more productive, but it's liberated my personal time so I can be at my best for the people I love. Maintaining discipline gives me freedom.

I have been able to strike a balance that allows me to be at my best when I'm on clinic and at home by scheduling and using my hush time effectively. I have time in my diary to reflect regularly and to ensure my career is heading in the right direction. Everything we decide to do is also a decision not to do everything else so we need to make sure we prioritise only those tasks that are going to help us fulfil our purpose and move forward.

Only you can decide what is important to you, but I hope you can do so by using your purpose and direction. Having found the right balance and structured our lives to maintain a high level of performance, we now need to focus our attention on our chosen profession and what it is within dentistry we can do to thrive.

# 10

# Don't Stop Me Now

## Queen

### *How to thrive in dentistry*

"How long will you wait before you demand the best of yourself, and trust reason to determine what is best?"
**Marcus Aurelius**

While doing my research for this book I spoke to over 60 people working in dentistry, including clinicians, dental care professionals, dental technicians, business coaches and even a select few people from outside the profession. I asked them why they love what they do and I discovered many recurring themes. The answers people gave me can be found at the back of this book, but to summarise, most people found a real passion in their careers when they learned how to truly connect with the people around them and when they started to feel like they were making a meaningful difference in people's lives. If we want to make a real difference for our patients, we need to use our purpose to help us decide which direction we want our career to take. We need to develop our skills through effective learning and deliberate practice and we need to build the right environment around ourselves.

Dentistry is not an easy profession to work in and this is one of the reasons I love it. Most people don't have the right combination of the hard and soft skills that are needed to build trusting relationships with patients, diagnose and prevent or treat their problems. The difficulty of the job means we need to make investments in ourselves throughout our careers to keep improving so we can always be at our best.

"The best time to plant a tree was twenty years ago, the second-best time is now."
**Chinese Proverb**

It's tempting to wait for a future date, usually one that's based on the earth's orbit around the sun, before we make a significant change but if we have to wait for this arbitrary time in the future, the change isn't important enough to us. Important changes are made immediately. Dare I say, by reading this book, maybe you've already started. That said, even with the best of intentions, a purpose, a direction and the right mindset, it can be difficult to know where to begin. How do I implement these wonderful habits that will incrementally improve my life? Where do I find the best CPD? How can I get the right job in the right place where I can thrive?

It starts with the introspection that formed the first few chapters of this book. What really matters most to me? Where am I now and in which direction do I want my career to go? Once we've spent the time establishing what matters to us, we can start taking small steps, building small habits on our journey. There is no perfect first step, the place to start for everyone is different but it usually begins with making the changes that we can make today, making small changes that are easy to implement.

## A Thousand Words

If I had to suggest a single place to start for any clinician, it would be in investing in a camera. There is no more powerful tool for reflecting on the work we've done than being able to see it blown up on a high-definition screen. Pictures allow us to reflect on each step of the process in graphic detail. Often when I've completed a long treatment my eyes are tired, I've been staring at a small segment of the mouth for so long that I can't focus any more. It's only when I review the photographs that I can see where I can improve. I may have just spent fifteen minutes shaping the perfect molar fissure pattern in composite, only to see on a photo that I've left a huge flash of composite around a buccal cusp. How long would that have been left and what would be the damage if I hadn't taken the photo? How many more times would I have repeated that mistake before noticing it?

When I'm undertaking more advanced treatments, I

take photographs of every step from the assessment to the annual reviews, in every single case. I've not placed a single implant that I don't believe I could have done a little better in one way or another and when I reflect on the photos, I can often identify the critical moment during treatment when I could have done a little better. It's only by reflecting using these photographs that I've been able to improve my skills, otherwise, I'd still be hitting golf balls in the dark, with no idea where they're going.

Like any new skill, it takes a bit longer at first to take these pictures. Now though, taking a photo makes very little difference to my treatment time but it has a huge impact on the quality of my care. I don't even take many of my own photos, the camera is always set up, ready on the worktop on the right settings and it's so easy to use that my young kids can take a perfect smile photo (yes, I have tested this). The photos I take don't just help me reflect, I use them with my patients, to communicate with my lab tech, when I'm lecturing and as part of my clinical notes.

## Effective Learning

I was very fortunate to have Professor Simon Wright as my mentor in my formative years placing dental implants, before he became a Professor or received his MBE. Simon is a remarkable surgeon with a career-long dedication to improving his skills and improving patient safety both in his own practice and by lecturing internationally on the subject of human factors in dentistry. He was also a very supportive mentor and he has probably had a bigger influence on my career than any other dentist. Through his experience of thousands of implant placements, he gained an understanding of the best way to treat each patient and in time, an understanding of which steps were essential in which cases and which steps could be bypassed to speed up a patient's journey.

One such step is uncovering a dental implant that has been left to heal submucosally, usually, this is a standalone appointment, with a subsequent appointment to take an impression or scan of the implant with healed soft tissues around it. In some situations, he would uncover the implant and take an impression at the same appointment, saving an extra appointment and giving his patient a fixed tooth back a couple of weeks quicker. Of course, I saw him doing this and I copied him, though I did so without first understanding when and why he was doing this. This worked perfectly when he mentored me because he made sure I only did it in cases where it was appropriate, but I failed to learn when it wasn't the right decision.

"We don't rise to the level of our expectations we fall to the level of our training."
**Archilochus**

When I started to restore implants independently, I came unstuck. After following the steps above, I came to fit an implant crown and the titanium abutment margin was exposed above the gum causing a big aesthetic problem. It happened because I'd failed to account for the soft tissue remodelling that happens after uncovering an implant, something that often is very minor, but can be very significant, as it was in this case. Fortunately, no harm was done but it taught me an important lesson about understanding the treatment I'm providing before trying to skip important steps. The 'Simon says' defence is completely inappropriate when our treatment hasn't turned out the way we had intended.

One of the issues in this situation was that my mentor was so far ahead of me in terms of knowledge and skill that I was unable to comprehend everything he was doing. The same problem can make choosing our CPD, we can be drawn in by the most glamorous courses, taught by immensely skilled clinicians, but we'll struggle to gain much from them if they're too far beyond our current skill and understanding.

Jumping around from one course to another is expensive, both in terms of time and money. I have amassed over two thousand hours of verifiable CPD since I qualified as a dentist, often by doing just this, meandering from one course to another without any real purpose. In contrast, taking the time to reflect on which specific areas we want to develop allows us to select the courses that are going to be the greatest benefit to us and our patients.

We need to choose courses that are at the right level for our ability, so we can implement our newly learned skills immediately, before we forget how to use them. I've been guilty in the past of attending courses that are teaching techniques that are well above my skill level. All that happened was I made a ton of notes about subjects I had little comprehension of, and I'd leave wanting to do everything but without the confidence or ability to see it through.

I discovered my passion for implant dentistry early in my career and the first step I took was to shadow as many procedures as I could, to gain some understanding of how dental implants work in the real world. I was helped, of course, by breaking my arm, but I chose not only to shadow the dentists in my practice but to observe as many other clinicians as I could. The most valuable experiences were those times when I watched someone who wasn't too far ahead of me, someone who remembers how it feels to be on the bottom rung of the ladder doing things I could envisage myself doing in the not too distant future.

I set about arming myself with as much knowledge on dental implants by reading journals and books which gave me a big head start before undertaking any formal training. Before going on an implant course, I also started to practise my basic surgical skills, like flap design and suturing on my normal clinics. Extra shifts on emergency clinics were a great way to seek out difficult extractions and gain exposure to more surgical dentistry.

I began looking for patients who may be suitable for my first implant case. The ideal patient never arrives just after we've been on the course and so it makes all the difference to find a patient with whom we have a good rapport before our new journey starts. This way, we can be ready to get the most difficult first treatment under our belt, with appropriate mentorship, while all that learning is still fresh in our memory. This is how to truly get value from our education, it is anything but a passive process. Effective learning only happens when we engage with the process, instead of just hunting for another certificate.

Even with this preparation, it can be difficult to change how we work. It takes a lot of energy to break old habits, form better ones and implement new skills, so it helps to make it as easy as possible. For many years I would leave a course inspired and energised about all the new things I could do, only to find that several months later, I'd failed to implement anything I'd learned. I now make a simple list of three things that I want to implement following any learning experience. Keeping this list confined to the three most important things focuses my efforts on making the greatest impact on my practice. This is far more effective than having pages of notes littered with small gains that get lost in time.

The best way to master a subject is to teach it and so when I've been on a course, I will go back to my practice and teach the team around me what I've learned as well. Not only does this consolidate my learning, but it involves the team more in a patient's care and it helps them to understand why we're changing the way we're doing things. Change isn't always easy, and some people struggle more than others, particularly when a change has been forced upon them. Showing the team what I've learned and why it will help our patients also helps them to hold me to account for implementing it. If everyone in my environment is committed to the change, it makes it much easier for me to maintain my habits. Implementing our learning is as simple as forming new habits and this is the foundation of making meaningful long-lasting improvements to our lives.

> "The more disciplined your environment is, the less disciplined you need to be."
> **James Clear**

We can make improvements to our home or work environments at any time but sometimes we have to change our environment altogether to move forward. For us to perform at our best, we need to be in an environment that supports our development. Being in the right environment doesn't necessarily mean having the best equipment and the biggest room to work in, the people who surround us are far more important. Being part of a team who wants to improve and grow is vital if we are to keep developing.

# A Career in Dentistry

There are hundreds of different careers within dentistry and a large proportion of us will choose to be part of one of the most important and most challenging which is that of primary general dental care. Specialist dentists often take the plaudits as the ones at the peak of the profession but it's the specialist generalist who needs to have the most extensive range of knowledge and skills to be at their best. I love providing dental implant treatment for my patients, but I also love the variety of treatments I can provide as a general dentist too. Treating anxious patients can be incredibly challenging, yet there are few more gratifying experiences than rebuilding a petrified patient's confidence. The same is true of treating children, often difficult, but it can be great fun and very rewarding. The revelry of completing a full rehabilitation or the gore of 'gum-gardening'.

There's so much more on offer than general dentistry though, from community to hospital consultancy, specialism in a single practice or peripatetic work. Then there's the myriad of non-clinical roles in research and education, the possibilities are endless, and that's just for dentists. How then do we even start to think about which direction we want to take?

Most people starting their careers in dentistry now will face the prospect of forty years in the profession. This opens up a world of opportunity with time to explore and enjoy the variety of careers on offer. We don't need to decide which path to take straight away. I know many dentists who have completed dental implant courses, even finishing a master's degree before deciding that implant dentistry isn't for them. That's not to say this is an effective way to approach your development but to highlight that we're not restricted to a single path no matter what our level of education.

Like Columbus setting off to circumnavigate the globe, we begin with exploration, perhaps with a direction in mind, and we may be surprised about where we find ourselves. My journey began shadowing many different dentists from all walks of dentistry to find what I was passionate about. Not only did this give me an insight into what aspects of dentistry I found fascinating, but I learned a wide range of skills and techniques, particularly from people on career pathways that I knew I didn't want to pursue. When we focus so narrowly on a single philosophy we lose the ability to cross-pollinate ideas from divergent schools of thought inside and outside of the dentosphere.

In a world of immediacy, where everything is available at the click of a mouse, it's easy to believe that everything we want should be available to us right now, including what we presently think of as our dream job. But the perfect job doesn't exist, there are always compromises and by dreaming of the greener grass, we can fail to live in the moment. We don't enjoy what we have, and we don't develop our skills as we wait for something better to come along. That dream job is an outcome and we can't control our outcomes. All we can do is improve our process, invest in ourselves, develop our skills and be ready to take the opportunities when they arrive.

The best jobs are usually taken before a job advert gets posted and the best clinicians are often offered the best jobs before they start looking. Be under no illusion that these clinicians will have almost certainly run the long yards to create these opportunities for themselves. They'll have worked the on-calls, the unsociable hours, and worked in areas of high need and low appreciation.

They've also not waited for the opportunities to come to them, but they've taken steps to get themselves noticed by the people who may be able to provide them with an environment in which to flourish. They'll have also taken steps to be able to demonstrate their commitment to patient care, personal development and teamwork.

A professional portfolio, for instance, can allow us to show a sample of our work, but more important than this, it shows our commitment to critically reflect on our work. Our portfolio, therefore, is not a highlights reel of our most superficially aesthetic work, but a chance to demonstrate our ability to reflect on our strengths and weakness, our desire to learn and our commitment to keep improving.

We also need to understand our values and those of the practice where we work, or want to work. By now, I hope you understand the power of your purpose and its importance in helping you grow. Every team and business will also have their values and purpose, whether they're articulated or not and aligning our values provides the best environment for the individual and the practice to grow. Each clinician is but a small part of a larger team, even in the smallest practices. The best team members are the ones who help to raise up the people around them and these individuals who contribute the most to the team, are usually the ones who ultimately get the most out in the end.

Early in my career, I found myself in a job where I didn't feel the principal dentist's values aligned with my own. I didn't feel supported and I wasn't able to do my best work. With the benefit of hindsight, there are many things I could have done to improve the situation. I was unreceptive to ideas different from the views I held and the notions of buying some of my own equipment or taking the lead in trying to build stronger relationships with the people around me were completely foreign concepts. I also failed to consider things from the principal's position. As an associate, this was just another job for me, one in which I wanted to do my best for the patients and my development but one that I could leave whenever I wanted. To the principal, the practice, the team and the patients are their life and their family. In offering me a job, he'd invited me to be a part of that family and he was concerned for the wellbeing of everyone he felt responsible for. As an associate, I wanted to be trusted and given the freedom to provide the best care I could for my patients, but these liberties must be earned, not assumed.

The experienced dentist turned owner wants the best for their team and their patients, and it's not easy for them to do what feels like abdicating their responsibilities to give a clinician the freedom they often desire, particularly, when the associate is as inexperienced as I was. When we have demonstrated our trustworthiness, reliability, team ethic, clinical proficiency and a drive to go above and beyond to help our patients and the practice, even when it doesn't have an immediate pay-off for us, then, and only then, may we start to reap the rewards of trust and clinical freedom.

# Coda

| Three steps to mastery |
|---|
| 1. Use your purpose and reflection about your own strengths and weaknesses to find courses that are appropriate to your skill level. Remember, we succeed, not because we don't have any weaknesses, but because we play to our strengths. |
| 2. Take photos, use them to reflect on your work and start to build a portfolio geared towards growth. |
| 3. Reflect on your education and identify three things you've learned that you can implement in your practice immediately. |

It's cheesy, but I believe dentistry is my calling. It's not a profession that just anyone can thrive in and this is one of the reasons I love it. With this challenge comes an acceptance that we must keep learning throughout our careers, and this is far more effective if we take the time to reflect on our current ability and seek out appropriate areas for development.

We can maximise our growth by making sure we engage in effective learning, not jumping from one course to the next, but seeking those opportunities that are best suited to our abilities right now and ensuring we implement our training. The best opportunities are always the ones that require a level of skill that's a little bit higher than we currently have. It takes us just far enough out of our comfort zone to reach a state of flow, but not so far that we're working beyond our competency.

The best time to start making improvements is right now but we don't have to do everything immediately. A long and fruitful career in dentistry is one filled with diversity which will bring new challenges and opportunities to keep our passion burning as we evolve.

I started this chapter by explaining that most people who are passionate about their work, feel this way because of the connections they make with the people they're privileged to help. It's the relationships we develop with our patients that can spark the passion in our careers and in order to make this connection, we need to focus on the single most important part of dentistry, communication.

# 11

# Transmission

## Joy Division

### *How to communicate effectively*

"Every human creature is constituted to be that profound
secret and mystery to every other."
**Charles Dickens**

Any chimp can be trained to drill a hole and fill it, the
bulk of what we consider routine dentistry is, in reality,
not a great deal more than intra-oral carpentry. Our ability
to diagnose and plan is often what separates good
dentists and great ones from a professional perspective,
but it's our communication skills that will define us as
good or bad dentists in the eyes of our patients. To be
able to truly help our patients, we must be able to form
trusting relationships with them. We must create an

environment where they can be open with us, so we can understand what is important to them. It's only once we recognise our patient as a person that we can begin to help them in a meaningful way. Without building this connection, our patients won't trust us and without trust, we can't help them.

Learning to communicate effectively with our patients is the hardest skill to master within dentistry, made worse as we dentists are typically not the archetypal socialite. The demand for academic acumen to get into university means that we are mostly left-brain thinkers, logicians and neurotics. In school, prospective dentists tend to be book-smart but they're often not high on the popularity scale, with a distinct tendency towards introversion. These traits are great for focusing on our studies, but not so useful for talking to strangers.

I remember my sessions on clinic at uni, sitting around for what felt like hours, in a deafening silence waiting for a tutor to check my little occlusal composite before discharging the patient. I knew that I should be able to have a conversation with my patient in this time, but I didn't know where to start. I found it hard to have the most superficial conversation, not helped by the introvert label I'd given myself.

Marisa's studies for her diploma in counselling and psychotherapy involved a lot of self-directed learning, on her own, off campus. At the time, I was plying my trade in a busy NHS practice, working on my communication skills, and trying to develop rapport with more than forty patients in a day. By the end of the day, I would be wiped out. Our starkly different daily grinds meant that Marisa, having spent all day alone, would want to spend much of the evening talking and I would want to curl up in bed without speaking or hearing another word. It put a strain on our relationship, I was spending so much of my energy trying to connect with my patients, that I had nothing left for her at the end of the day. Engaging our patients on a meaningful level is emotionally expensive and this can have an impact beyond our nine-to-five. The good news is that just like physical exercise, the more you do, the easier it becomes.

"We are not in the coffee business serving people, but in the people business serving coffee"
**Howard Schultz, CEO of Starbucks**

We are in the caring for people business, it just so happens that fixing teeth is one of the ways we do this. Most people choose a career in healthcare because they want to help people, but we can lose sight of this ambition with a myopia on what's happening within the mouth, rather than to whom the mouth is attached. The onus is on us to put our patients at ease and earn their trust and the only way we can do this is through communication. I still cringe thinking of some of my early attempts at making conversation with my patients but that's ok because I was learning a new skill and like any skill, it takes time to develop. I still don't always find it easy, but I can usually find some common ground, unrelated to dentistry when I meet a patient for the first time.

# Empathic Listening

Most people are nervous when they make their first visit to a new dental practice and taking the time to get to know someone, just a little bit, before interrogating them about their oral health will put them at ease. Good communication is the only way we can make meaningful connections with our patients. If we can take the time to do this at the start of an appointment, by the time it comes to talking teeth, our patients will usually be more relaxed and open about their genuine concerns. We cannot fake this relationship, there are no gimmicks or magic phrases that will convince every patient to trust us, nor should there be. The most difficult things are the most rewarding which is why again I remind you that most of the dentists I spoke to love what they do, based on the connections that they make with their patients.

When the world started to turn again in 2020 after the first coronavirus lockdown, we started to return to work. Due to the need for donning and doffing PPE and fallow times every appointment was made a bit longer. As things slowly returned to normal we stopped vigilantly policing the amount of time a patient was in the practice. I would often find I had more time than I needed for my appointments. Rather than grabbing an extra cup of tea, I used this time to talk to my patients. Sometimes we'd talk about teeth, often about COVID, but frequently we'd talk about music, food, books, sport or family. I developed a deeper connection with each patient and after an extra five minutes of talking about anything, my patients would often bring the conversation back around to their teeth and ask me again about filling a gap or what could be done to make their teeth healthier. Rather than me nagging my patients to floss, they were asking me what they could do to improve the health of their teeth. Once my patients felt that I would listen and understand them, they would open up about being embarrassed about the colour of their teeth. By giving my patients the opportunity to talk, they give me the opportunity to better help them.

Our patients are often too scared to tell us about these concerns, many don't want to feel vain and are often embarrassed about wanting to spend money on themselves for what they perceive as luxuries, like cosmetic dental treatment. In the words of one of my friends, 'I want my teeth to be whiter, but I don't want anyone to know I've had them whitened.' On the face of it, that sounds ridiculous, but consider what he's really saying here. He wants to have confidence in his smile, he wants his teeth to look and feel clean, bright and healthy. He's not vain, so he was a bit embarrassed about saying this to me, but he wants to feel confident in himself. By dedicating a little more time to the person in front of us, we can build that trust, and this allows our patients to talk to us about what really matters to them.

"When dealing with people, let us remember we are not dealing with creatures of logic. We are dealing with creatures of emotion, creatures bristling with prejudices and motivated by pride and vanity."
**Dale Carnegie**

Some people seem to have a natural ability to connect with people quickly, they can walk into a room and strike up a conversation with anyone. For the rest of us, it takes time and deliberate practice to develop the skill. By taking the time to understand who the person behind the teeth is, we will also gain an insight into what their motivation for dental treatment is, whether it's simply health, or in preparation for a big occasion or any significant life event. Once we understand who our patient is, we can start to help them in more meaningful ways. If we can demonstrate to our patients that we're going to listen empathically and without judgement, our patients are more likely to open up fully about themselves so we can understand how best to help them.

Empathic listening goes beyond processing the words that we hear. It is about being in tune with our interlocutor, understanding their emotions and reflecting what they've expressed back to them in our own way. In doing so, we demonstrate not only that we heard the words they said, but we understand what they mean and the emotions that drive them. Empathic listening is difficult to master because we can only live our lives from our own perspective, drawing on our own experiences. What works for us in one situation is often not in any way applicable to anyone else, and what we believe is the right treatment for a particular tooth, may be the wrong solution for the person it's attached to.

We cannot feel exactly as our patients do because we have not lived their experiences, however, we can accept their emotions and show them that we appreciate that these things are important to them. Empathy is about understanding the feelings of someone else and when we show a desire to do this, even if we don't always get it exactly right, our patients will feel our care instead of just hoping it's there. When we take the time to understand our patients and their motivations, we can work with them to find the best solution. When their treatment is complete, we are more likely to have a happy patient because we've worked with them and their emotions and not in spite of them.

Part of listening to our patients is also trying to understand what their expectations are of their treatment, whether they want our help to restore health and function, aesthetics, phonetics or for psychological reasons. Most patients seeking cosmetic treatment will have an end result in mind and often, perhaps due to what they see in the media, this can be entirely unrealistic. Again, we need to listen first, we need to understand what it is our patient wants and why they want it.

"Seek first to understand, then to be understood."
**Stephen Covey**

We must listen without judgement and show our patients we have understood their needs. It can be very easy to silence a patient by jumping in to correct them when they tell us something factually incorrect or unrealistic, but by stopping the conversation we are showing them that we're no longer willing to listen to them. We all encounter patients who believe their gums bleed because they brush too hard, but dismissing their views out of hand is only likely to embarrass your patient and close the conversation down. By empathically listening and showing our patients that we've understood their perspective, they are far more likely to engage with what we say to them.

# Cultivating Clarity

We communicate primarily not through the words we use but the way we use them, our tone of voice and body language. Good friends do this subconsciously with each other because they share empathy, they often speak and act similarly. If we want to understand our patients, we must try to empathise with them, to put ourselves in their position. Paying attention to their body language, the pace and tone of their speech and reflecting this back to them when we repeat what they've told us, shows our patients that we've paid attention to them and care about what they've said. It also helps us develop empathy with them, allowing us to find a deeper connection than just consuming their words.

The same is true when we are communicating how we can help our patients, we will be better understood if we can tailor our message to the person we're trying to reach. We speak to a young child differently from an adult, but we sometimes fail to communicate effectively by talking to all adults in the same way. Failure in this regard will not only likely leave our patients confused or scared, but if they choose to go ahead with treatment, could invalidate any consent we feel has been given. By way of example and admittedly with a sweeping generalisation, fellow healthcare professionals like lots of detail about their treatment, they want to know every nuance of how each procedure will be performed. If we give this level of information to an anxious patient, we might never see them again. We must give enough information for the patient to provide informed consent, but this doesn't mean everyone needs or wants the same level of detail.

Varying how we deliver this information is also important. VARK learning describes how there are four styles of learning, visual, auditory, read/write, and kinaesthetic, we are all a blend of each, but each person usually has a dominant learning style.

Visual learners need to see the problem to understand it. The most effective way to do this is by showing a patient a picture or intra-oral scan of their teeth, perhaps complimented by a diagram for problems that are going on under the surface.

Auditory learners understand best when we discuss their treatment with them. Using appropriate metaphors is an effective way of making abstract dental problems more concrete for our patients. For example, when communicating the importance of treating gum disease before cosmetic treatment, I explain that there's no point in fixing the roof of a house if the foundations aren't strong.

Read/write learners will benefit greatly from a written summary or treatment plan letter which they can digest in their own time.

Kinaesthetic learners show a much deeper understanding if they can get hold of a demonstration model and explore the problem for themselves, with some guidance.

It's not practical to undertake extensive questionnaires to ascertain each patient's learning style, so we must present important information in a variety of ways to all patients. In doing this, we can gauge our patient's level of engagement and further tailor our message to the individual.

The human body is incomprehensibly complex, we can never deal in absolutes and there are an infinite number of possible options in any situation. When communicating options to our patients, it's important to keep things simple, the best way to put someone off doing something, even if we know it will help them, is to make the problem too complicated. As a rule, I try to limit the treatment options I give to my patients to three, the two best interventions, plus the option and consequences of doing nothing. We can explain why certain alternatives are not appropriate, but I have found that by offering more than three options, I only confuse an already complicated situation. These options should be communicated based on our understanding of the specific patient's concerns, their age, general health, likely compliance and a myriad of other patient-specific factors. We must be clear about the benefit of our recommended option in the context of what our patient has told us is important to them.

We must be clear on realistic expectations about all treatments from the outset, not only in terms of the appearance but also the likelihood of discomfort, the need for remedial treatment, how long the treatment is likely to take and how long it will last. If we don't feel we can achieve the level of treatment that our patient is expecting, and they're unwilling to change their expectations, then we must not treat them. Early in my career, I feared I would put my patients off a perfectly reasonable treatment and so I tended to underplay the risks and overpromise the benefits. I was caught out a few times when things didn't turn out exactly as I'd planned or a patient had more post-operative discomfort than I'd expected.

Now I do the opposite. I give all my patients the worst-case scenario, with reassurance that it is the worst-case scenario, that they're likely to expect swelling and pain after an extraction for instance. Whilst I never want my patients to have any pain, if they do have significant post-operative discomfort, it's manageable they were expecting it. If, on the other hand, our patient doesn't have any pain, they're likely to be delighted as things are much better than they'd thought. Neither scenario has anything to do with my technical ability, it's simply managing a patient's expectations. The patient expecting no pain will feel far worse with a niggle, than a patient expecting agony.

Next, we need to discuss the costs and it has taken me many years to feel comfortable having this conversation. I have grown in confidence in discussing money, firstly, by understanding how much it costs to keep a dental practice fully staffed and open all day every day, but also by valuing myself and my skills. Ashley Latter's book Don't Wait For the Tooth Fairy helped me hugely in this regard. In it, Ashley tells the story of Pablo Picasso, who was dining at a New York restaurant when he was asked by a fan to draw a picture for her. Reaching for a napkin, Picasso quickly sketched the waiter before handing it to her and asking for $10,000 in payment. 'But it took you less than five minutes' she exclaimed, to which Picasso replied 'no madam, it took me a lifetime.' The value of being able to provide a service is not tied up solely in the amount of time spent, but in the years of training and dedicated practice to get there.

When I left university, I'd spent five years living on £9,000 per year, including rent and tuition fees. At that time, £2,000 for a dental implant was an exorbitant amount. I couldn't imagine spending that much money on a single tooth. I even felt uncomfortable telling my patients they needed an NHS crown at £198. I felt like I was being the archetypal rip-off dentist because I had no idea how much it cost to run a dental practice and I had no sense of my worth. When I imagined working as a dentist, helping people, and fixing their teeth, I never considered I'd have to have awkward conversations about money and I had absolutely no training on the subject.

I've learned in time that these issues surrounding money belong to me and not my patients. It costs money to provide any dental treatment and it costs more money to provide higher-quality care. I have invested thousands of pounds in developing my skills and expertise to be able to provide the best care I can for my patients. Patients know and understand these things better than we do and it's not for us to deny a patient a valid treatment option because we think it's too expensive for them. In fact, it would be remiss for us to do so. It's not our job to decide whether our patients can afford a certain treatment, it's very much our job to make sure they can make a fully informed decision about what is best for them.

I conclude the conversation with a summary of the benefits of the treatment I believe is the best for them and why, again relating this back to their concerns. 'I think the best option for you is to place two dental implants and a bridge over the top. This will give you fixed teeth back so you can get rid of your denture and start enjoying eating your steak and chips again.' Or 'by replacing the old crowns at the front of your mouth, you will be able to smile with confidence again, without worrying that people are looking at the dark lines near the gums.' By relating the treatment to what our patient has told us is important to them we show them we've listened and we're trying to find a solution that works for them, rather than taking a one-size-fits-all approach.

By taking the time to listen, understand and connect with our patients, not only do we build empathy and trust, we can provide better solutions for them as people and not just teeth. We can tailor our message back to them in a way that allows them to understand their treatment. This is vitally important for our patients to be able to give valid consent and it means we can begin to help people, rather than fixing holes.

# Coda

| Three steps to mastery |
|---|
| 1. Understand that it's the people that are at the heart of what we do, not the teeth. |
| 2. Communication begins with empathic listening, understanding our patients needs and desires and demonstrating that we've heard them. |
| 3. Communicating how we can help must be bespoke to each patient, to help them understand the information we give and how it relates to the things they've told us are important to them. |

The most caring and passionate people in dentistry understand that they're not in the business of fixing teeth, but the business of helping people, fixing teeth is just one of the ways we get to do this. No matter what our role is, everything we do in dentistry revolves around the people we are able to care for. We can choose to focus on filling holes and maybe we'll get paid well enough for doing so, but it's less fulfilling and unlikely to sustain a career. I don't just fill holes in teeth, I help restore my patient's confidence in their oral health, so they can live their lives without fearing the next broken tooth or abscess. I don't just provide tooth whitening, I help a father smile at his daughter's wedding. I don't just fill gaps with dental implants, I help foodies enjoy a proper meal without the fear of their teeth falling out.

In school, I always enjoyed maths, yet most of my

maths lessons, and dare I say teachers, were dull. The way my A-Level teacher, John, taught maths was different though. He wasn't just there to collect his pay and go home, I could see his passion for the subject and his students. When it came to parents' evening, John said something that I'll never forget, 'Karl is great at maths, I'm sure you don't need me to tell you that, but he's not a maths robot, he's got a fantastic personality. He's funny, he's warm and he's a pleasure to have in my class.' John was the first and only teacher that made me feel like I was more than just an exam mark at the end of the year. I loved those lessons and I thrived in that environment.

"People will forget what you said, people will forget what you did, but people will never forget how you made them feel."

**Maya Angelou**

It's nearly twenty years since John taught me for a single year in college and yet I've never forgotten the way he made me feel. It's not just about the words we say or the care we provide, but the way we listen, and the way we take the time to understand. By building meaningful connections with our patients, we can help them in ways that go beyond fixing teeth and this is the very heart of finding a passion in dentistry.

Dentistry is far from a solo enterprise though. Even with the best relationships with our patients, we can't do it alone. When I describe dentistry as being about the people, it's not just the patients, but the colleagues and team around me that make it so special.

# 12
# Join Together
## The Who

### *How to flourish in a community*

"Everything in existence takes its colour from the average hue of our surroundings."
**H.G. Wells - The Island of Doctor Moreau**

Evolution is a glacial process. We are the same, biologically speaking, as the Homo Sapiens who roamed the earth 30,000 years ago and yet our world couldn't be more different. We no longer need to forage for every morsel of food, I'm typing on my MacBook Pro while my smart oven is cooking my dinner and I can track that my next delivery is seven stops away. We have nuclear power, quantum physics and more information than you could read in a lifetime about both available at the push of a button. How can we be genetically identical to those first humans and yet occupy a world so incomprehensibly different to the one we first evolved into?

This intellectual and cultural evolution was brought about by our ability to communicate, initially in small tribes, and now globally. As our communication systems have become quicker and further reaching, the rate of change around us has accelerated. The acquisition of knowledge has evolved from relying entirely on our elders to pass down knowledge by word of mouth, to the infinite resource of the internet where we can access anything, published by anyone, anywhere, at any time. Of course, the challenge remains in choosing which information to trust. The disclaimer to this book is that I've presented to you my opinions based on my own experiences, mistakes and biases. They're shared with the best of intentions, but it's up to you to decide which parts you want to apply to your own life.

I have always been receptive to anyone offering their time to offer guidance and by listening to a range of views, I can choose what to apply to my own life. It's in choosing which advice to follow that the challenge lies. We enjoy hearing things that validate our preconceptions and we feel uncomfortable with opinions dissonant with our worldview. Our instinctive response is to dismiss such views out of hand, and this stifles our development. Nobody forms an opinion without having a justification for it, so even when we vehemently disagree, it helps to be receptive to their view and to try to understand why they feel as they do, rather than seeking to immediately oppose their position. By building a network of people around us with diverse experiences, different roles and divergent opinions from our own, we can develop a more comprehensive view of the world, hopefully, one that is a little less prejudiced.

It's the people we choose to surround ourselves with that shape who we are. I have played badminton for most of my life on and off. My ability has improved over the years with practice, as you would expect, but the swiftest improvements have come when I play with people who are just a little bit better than me. Whether we like it or not, our lives are shaped by our environment, it helps therefore, to be surrounded by people who want to grow and develop like us. It's not just about surrounding ourselves with the most technically skilled clinicians, but being around people with the right mindset. People who aren't afraid to be honest with us, to contradict us or support us depending on the situation.

We're not just here to support each other on this journey of growth however, we're here to support each other when skies are grey. Dentistry can be an isolating profession, stuck in the same four walls day-in, day-out, but with a strong network around us, we can be present for each other. Even those people at the top of their game have bad days, treatments that don't go well, unhappy patients or times when they feel depressed or anxious for no good reason. We all need a shoulder to lean on at times and building a network isn't just about pushing each other up the ladder, it's the safety net to catch us when we fall too. This safety net isn't just for us, we get to be there for other people too. We may be fortunate to find such a network within the four walls of our daily practice, but this isn't the case for the majority of people. Once we leave the highly social environment of university we can lose touch with the rest of the profession unless we choose to actively seek out these connections.

It would be nice if we could wake up on our first day of a new job and instantly be connected to our new team and all the clinicians in our local area. It takes time to find the right people to fill our network though and we have to look for opportunities to meet new people. Courses and conferences are great places to meet colleagues, particularly events like study clubs that offer an opportunity to mix in a relaxed environment. Joining local dental committees and getting involved in associations is also a fantastic way to connect with people who want to make a difference in the profession, and it also allows us to give something back. It's easy to mix with people like ourselves, but it's more enriching to connect with people that challenge our preconceptions.

# Collaboration

Queen dominated the mid-70s rock scene but in the early 80's they lost their edge. Their creativity seemed to dry up and what resulted were some mediocre albums with the odd hit amongst the filler. Whilst they never officially split up, around 1983 each band member started to pursue solo projects, diversifying their surroundings, heading in different musical directions and enriching their tapestry. When they came back together, they produced The Works, one of my favourite Queen albums. The broadening of their horizons and the collaborations outside of the confines of their familiar environment helped them to revitalise the band. What followed was Queen's legendary LiveAid performance, selling out back-to-back nights at Wembley and then Freddie's final show to 120,000 people at Knebworth.

It's this very spirit of collaboration that we can incorporate into our own lives. One area of dentistry that keeps me stimulated and engaged on a daily basis is problem-solving. Every patient is different, as is every tooth, and so the solutions are rarely one-size fits all. We can assume that dentistry in its simplest form doesn't require a great deal of collaboration but even on the scale of individual teeth, there can be a multitude of treatment options. Ten dentists may have ten equally valid ways of managing a given problem and we don't have a crystal ball to tell us what is best for each specific patient, with any level of certainty. We view the problems we're presented with through our own lens, shaped by our own experiences and biases. Taking time out to canvas for different opinions can open our eyes to new or even old treatments that we may have never otherwise considered.

If we start to undertake more complex work with a dozen or more teeth to assess, diagnose, and evaluate treatment options for each, the possibilities become infinite. No single dentist can know the best solution in every given situation and it's only through collaboration with our colleagues, lab technicians, team, and patient that we can make the most complex treatment decisions.

An unexpected trend has emerged in my career, as my experience has grown, I find myself seeking out the opinions of others more frequently. The more I know, the more I realise I don't know. When I collaborate with other professionals, I find better solutions for my patients and I gain a deeper understanding of the gaps in my knowledge. There is an infinite amount of information which we do not know and learning to accept we have blind spots in our knowledge is the first step in minimising their impact. By working with clinicians with different training and different backgrounds you get different opinions and collectively you can come up with a more comprehensive plan than any individual could produce alone.

This collaboration can begin in-house for some, but for others, it may be video calls or group chats that can provide the necessary platform. Ad hoc support can be useful, but I have found booking regular sessions, usually tagged on to a lunchtime, dedicated to case discussions, the most beneficial. Wherever we garner this support, we need to ensure we're doing so in a safe, controlled environment, where we know we can trust the advice we're receiving, where people aren't afraid to speak up for fear of being chastised for proffering opinion or if they disagree with something. We have never lived in a better time for collaborating remotely, with access to clinicians across different specialities and even in different countries.

Through social media, we can take inspiration from what other dentists are sharing and be introduced to potentially better solutions to common and uncommon problems. Social media offers us an opportunity to connect with our patients and our colleagues like never before, to share a little more of ourselves and what we do to either help the right patients find us or help us connect with the right colleagues. It's also a great platform for disseminating information about courses or jobs, both of which often come with some validation from peers.

Many caveats come with the use of social media, however. When looking at presented cases we're viewing other peoples' highlights reels and this can be misleading. You only see what people want you to see, there's rarely any acknowledgement about the failure rates of treatments and you don't see the five similar cases that didn't turn out quite as well. The instant nature of before and afters can promote the idea that every treatment is completed quickly and effortlessly, and we certainly don't see the hours of training and practice by the clinician to develop their skills.

With an understanding of these limitations, we can use social media to take inspiration and connect with colleagues near and far. Alongside social media, podcasts are useful in providing insights into aspects of dentistry we may not be privy to elsewhere. These may pique our interest and encourage us to seek further education, or often, they can simply make us think and reflect on our practice and how we can improve the way we work. The best podcasts often also have a loyal following with groups of similarly passionate clinicians brought together on social media or messaging groups where the spirit of collaboration can thrive in a more protected environment than an open online forum. We can use this social sphere to complement our learning and help us develop our network and doing so will bring new opportunities to the fore.

# Mentors

With the empowerment that comes from being able to connect with anyone, comes the opportunity to learn from anyone at any time. I didn't have any family, or friends in the dental or medical fields before starting dental school and so I didn't naturally have anyone to follow other than the people I found myself around on my journey. I initially envied those who seemed to get a leg up on the career ladder through their dental heritage, but I soon embraced the luxury of choice. I didn't have a preordained path and I could choose who I wanted to learn from and which direction I wanted my career to take.

My exploration into career options in dentistry began by shadowing a clamour of clinicians and it was the implantologists who rose above the noise. I was fortunate to be in a practice where implants were already being placed, but from there I asked for their recommendations on other people who I could observe as well as asking lecturers on courses or even delegates who were a bit further along their journey.

Through shadowing, I saw the difference that implant treatments could make in someone's life, but it was the passion and care that I witnessed in these dentists that impelled me to dive into the rabbit hole. It was these same dentists that I reached out to for mentoring when I started taking my first tentative steps into restoring implants and then placing them myself. Each mentor has gifted something different and helped me to develop in ways that a single teacher couldn't do. More important than the surgical skills I saw, my mentors have inspired me by the way they communicate with their patients, the way they assess and plan their cases, their passion for helping others and their commitment to keep improving themselves. I still try to seek out opportunities to shadow colleagues today, to gain a different perspective or learn a new technique.

To benefit the most from mentoring we must also become good mentees. There's nothing more frustrating as a mentor than when someone asks you for help without having made any effort to find a solution themselves. It's ok to plan a case incorrectly, these hard yards of planning and exploration of an unfamiliar subject will prepare our brains for learning more effectively when presented with a better solution. In these moments, it's the process of learning that's important, not just the outcome of getting the details of this specific case right.

We also have to be open to receiving constructive feedback. I've never yet completed the perfect treatment in any aspect of dentistry, there's always something that could be done better and so even when things have gone well, we should always be ready for at least one area for improvement as we're learning. If we've trusted someone to mentor us, we have to be prepared to hear things that we don't want to hear, such as being told we're not ready to undertake a complex case or that we could have done something better. The best mentors will provide an environment where we can safely put one foot out of our comfort zone and then provide constructive feedback that enables us to do a little better next time.

It's because I feel so uplifted by the mentoring I've received that I have become a mentor myself. The most effective teachers I've had have challenged my thinking, pushed me to come up with solutions myself instead and allowed me to struggle just a bit during surgery to allow me to discover my strengths and weaknesses. They've given me the confidence to undertake treatments that are within my competency and highlighted the situations that were beyond me at the time. As a mentor, I try to inspire my mentees with that same passion that I saw in others in my earlier years and empower my students with the tools to safely continue their journeys. In order to mentor effectively, I feel I've had to raise my game again to have a deeper understanding of the care we're providing and to understand the clinicians I'm working with, how to assess their strengths and weaknesses and provide meaningful feedback.

I owe an enormous debt of gratitude to the hundreds of people working within dentistry that I've encountered in my career so far, some I'm proud to call my mentors, others are friends, many are both. My career has been shaped by the people I've encountered on my journey. I have progressed by emulating those people I admire and respect from their surgical skills to the smallest turn of phrase which has helped me communicate with my patients.

We can spend a great deal of time and money training to become better clinicians with the best mentors to help us. We can go on courses to develop our skills in communicating with our patients but we fail to see that the people that have the biggest impact on us and in turn us on them, are the ones we spend the most time with. We spend most of our clinical time in the same room with the same person on whom we're dependent in order to thrive. For me, this is the dental care professional I work with every day, but I also rely on the rest of the team inside and outside the practice including other dentists, nurses, cleaners, hygienists, therapists, front-of-house staff, lab techs, and many, many more.

## Teamwork

"A team is not a group of people who work together, but a group of people who trust each other."
**Simon Sinek**

We cannot function as dentists without working effectively within a team of people. To perform at our best, we need to form positive relationships with everyone around us and this is dependent on mutual trust and respect. If we fail to work effectively in a team then we have no hope of providing the best care for our patients. The trust our team places in us is founded on our integrity, our commitment to doing what we say we're going to do, being disciplined with our words and actions and adhering to our moral code. Understand though that this does not mean being infallible, quite the opposite, we need to show that we're flawed humans. This means allowing ourselves to be vulnerable with the people closest to us, acknowledging when we've made a mistake or spoken out of turn. Be assured that there are no quick fixes to building trust, trust is built over time and we need to show that we, in turn, are willing to trust others. Trust is about mutual respect, it never flows in one direction only.

"That which is not good for the swarm, neither is it good for the bee."
**Marcus Aurelius**

Being part of the team means acting in the best interests of the team, often putting the group's interests before our own. This might mean we need to take the responsibility of speaking to an irate patient, owning the problem and finding a solution, rather than deflecting blame. Integrating into a team means not being above changing the toilet roll or picking up the crisp packet dumped on the waiting room floor. Of course, you don't delegate the daily job of mopping hospital corridors to the brain surgeon, but if we want to reap the benefits of an efficient team, the whole team needs to know that everyone will contribute to the big and the small tasks when necessary. A team can provide belonging and security, two vital ingredients for us to thrive. With a collective growth mindset, we no longer need to do everything ourselves, we can each work to our strengths for the greatest collective impact.

A farmer needs hay to feed her animals. She has two choices, she can buy some from the neighbour's farm, or she can save a little money and grow her own. While she may save some money in the short-term, growing hay requires a large field which could be used much more effectively in rearing more animals. What's more, the hay she buys is likely to be better quality if it's grown by someone whose whole farm is dedicated to growing the best hay.

As dentists, we can choose to try and do everything ourselves, every treatment, every step of the patient's journey, or we can focus on the things we're great at. Not only does this allow us to maximise the time we spend in flow, working in our area of true passion, but we also maximise the skillsets of the team around us. Is a patient getting the best possible care if one dentist does everything, or would they be better served by a team of people, each with a special interest? A treatment coordinator, an endodontist, an oral health educator, and a therapist to name but a few. In this way, teams are always more impactful than individuals and they also serve to elevate the individuals beyond where they could reach alone. The best way to fulfil our purpose then is to become a valuable member of a team who wants to grow together.

The strongest teams will always have shared values and will be striving towards the same purpose. I had shared my purpose with the people around me a few years ago and it was met with support and warmth, but I knew they didn't share the same passion I had. Not long after sharing my purpose with the team around me, we were fortunate to have Chris Barrow leading some in-house training focused on overcoming the challenges within dentistry. He emphasised the value of getting to know our patients, who they are and what's important to them as individuals, in order to provide a 'Champions League' level service to the people we're privileged to care for. After what I'd felt was an inspiring day, Vicky, who'd nursed alongside me for a couple of years, turned to me and said 'I don't get it, when I go to the dentist I just want my teeth checked.' The next day, our patient Sue came for her review appointment and in one moment, completely changed Vicky's whole outlook.

A few weeks earlier, Sue was petrified of 'the dentist', ashamed of her teeth and barely able to enter the waiting room, let alone have any treatment. It was the first time Sue had visited a dental practice for over ten years following a bad experience and her embarrassment about the condition of her teeth, she hadn't smiled for ten years either. She lived in constant fear of anyone seeing her teeth, including dental professionals. This fear dominated her entire life, she didn't laugh when she was out with friends and she always ate alone. She hadn't been to a restaurant in many years for fear of people seeing her teeth. Sue's dilemma was that her son was about to get married and she wanted to be able to smile in the photos, something she could not do with her teeth in their present condition.

It took time for us to build her confidence, first by talking to her away from the dental chair and listening to her bad experiences, her anxieties and her urgency in now finding a solution. It had taken her so long to raise the courage to finally make an appointment that it was a matter of weeks before the wedding. By taking the time to talk with Sue, we were able to show her we understood her problem and build the trust she needed to let us look at her teeth and help her find a solution. After talking Sue through her sadly limited options, she decided that the best option for her was to take out the remaining upper teeth and have a full denture, a conclusion she had pretty much come to herself beforehand despite knowing she was far too young to have this done.

We were short on time to get her wedding ready, but the whole team understood what it meant to her. Vicky agreed to work into our lunches to help get it done and our lab managed to shorten their turnaround time too. On the day we took her final few teeth out and fitted the full dentures, Sue was still understandably petrified but we got through it.

She came back to her review appointment armed with photos from the big day, like most weddings, there were smiles all around but there was one smile bigger than the rest. Sue filled up as she told us what it meant to her, to be able to smile at her son's wedding. This of course set me off too. After Sue left the surgery, Vicky turned to me, removing her sodden mask and said 'Karl, I get it.'

Vicky has never quite been the same since that day. She never stops going the extra mile for patients, whether it's follow-up phone calls, working late or just being there for a patient who needs to talk. She needs no instruction, no encouragement, she understands the impact we can have on our patients and she's committed to helping them every day of her working life. We didn't even do anything spectacular here, just a denture, but one made as a team with care and compassion for a person, not just to fill the gaps in another mouth.

# Coda

| Three steps to mastery |
|---|
| 1. Build positive, mutually constructive relationships with the people close to you and in your wider network. |
| 2. Engage with mentors, colleagues and peers to provide better care than any individual can. |
| 3. Look to raise up the people around you and work for the benefit of the collective, not yourself. |

Dentistry is far from a solo enterprise, we can spend a lifetime on personal improvement and never get anywhere if we fail to engage the people around us. If we surround ourselves with the right people, not only can they provide a platform for us to develop further, we can all grow stronger together and collectively achieve more than any individual. Not only this, but the reciprocal nature of networks has allowed me to help others in difficult times, just as I have been supported.

It's never been easier to connect with colleagues either through a broader array of courses, study clubs and social media, but connecting is an active process, it doesn't happen by chance. By understanding the direction we want our careers to take and we can start to build a network of the right type of people inside and outside of dentistry to help us get there. Through the connections I've made and maintained, I've had the opportunity to become a mentor and not only has this allowed me to pay forward the generosity that has been shown to me but it's proved an experience that has greatly accelerated my own learning.

By dedicating energy to developing strong bonds with the team around me I've found my work infinitely more rewarding. The best teams have an unwritten bond wherein there is mutual support through thick and thin and the knowledge that individual accomplishments will always pale in comparison to the collective growth of the team. Being in a team we can achieve far more than any individual and we can make a greater difference to our patients, our community, maybe even the world. There's something special about seeing those around you flourish, even if that means them moving on to new opportunities, just as I hope the people who've helped me to be where I am today, know how much it means to have been able to grow with them.

# To the End
## Blur

I love being a dentist, but it hasn't always been this way. A career in dentistry may come with many difficulties but none are insurmountable and a passion for the profession is accessible to anyone willing to put in the time to find it. It's no secret that in any job, the people who do it best, are the ones that love what they do. The passion that comes from loving our work drives us to overcome the obstacles we face, rise to the challenges and ultimately become the best versions of ourselves that we can be.

Passion, like happiness or success, is an outcome, an abstract destination on a landscape that is constantly changing. Our process, however, is entirely within our control. Passion is the result of what we do every day, the habits we keep, our mindset and our self-care. It's the relationships we build and nurture with our patients and the people around us that empower us all to grow together.

Even with a passion and a love of my job, I'm not

immune to fluctuations in my mental wellbeing, though I'm learning to ride the waves of my emotions instead of trying to fight against them. I am stronger for having been through my episodes of low mood and I hope my experiences will empower others to reach out when they need support and provide the tools for everyone to support the people around them.

Anyone can be In The Loupe and find fulfilment in what they do. My love for dentistry has grown with an understanding of my purpose, which has laid the foundations for lifelong personal development. Nobody enters this world with a passion for fixing teeth but this is not what dentistry is about. A career in dentistry is an opportunity to help people with a unique skill set and an infinite potential for growth. It can afford us the work-life balance that, if applied correctly, can be the key to sustainable fulfilment throughout our careers. Remember that not everything has to be done with maximum efficiency, keep a little slack in the system. We need time to rest and reflect, and we need flexibility to take advantage of new opportunities however they present.

Life is about more than teeth, we must not be consumed by what goes on inside the mouth. We're in the business of helping people, it just so happens that fixing teeth is often part of the solution. It's the relationships we build and seeing that we can make a positive difference in the lives of those around us that has inspired my passion. This passion drives me to keep improving so I can better care for myself, my family, my colleagues and my patients.

# Why Do You Love Being in Dentistry?

I hope this epilogue inspires you with some passion from a range of people who I believe are In The Loupe. On these pages you'll find some wonderful people in a variety of roles across dentistry, some you may know and others you won't, but all have inspired me in one way or another.

There is a disclaimer to add to this section. I asked them all a very leading question but there's a caveat. Most people told me that while they love their careers in general, it's not always the case. There are good days and bad. We're not all in a permanent state of passion and happiness, but we feel we're part of a worthy career where overall, the positives outweigh the negatives.

With that in mind, I want you to absorb the enthusiasm of the people who've taken the time to contribute to this peroration, identify the common threads in their answers and be inspired to find your own passion so you too can be In The Loupe.

**Simon Wright** @icedentalinstitute
Dentistry to me is more than just a job, it is a vocation and it very much defines who I am. There is nothing that gives me more pleasure than when a patient tells me that I have changed their life, or given them their life back.

**Chris Barrow** @coachbarrow
I love working in dentistry because it has allowed me to join a priceless network of friends, colleagues, peers and clients - people who have generously shared with me their hopes and dreams, their anxieties and fears and many of whom have realised their own potential by changing other people's lives for the better in this wonderful business.

**Chiggs Patel** @dr.chiggs
I love meeting people and developing relationships. In how many other professions can you say you've given someone a dream smile? Patients value what you've given them and they become loyal to you.

**Vicky Holroyd** @missvikss88
I love being a dental nurse because in the words of Forrest Gump, patients 'are like a box of chocolates, you never know what you're going to get.' There is no better feeling than giving a patient their smile and their confidence back. Every day is a new day, a new challenge which keeps me interested, and just being able to help patients is the biggest reward.

**Neal Heaher** @drnealheaher
I started to really enjoy dentistry when I began to change people rather than just single teeth.

**Amit Patel** @amitspecialistinperiodontics

I started to love dentistry when I found myself surrounded by people who would push me to be better and I started to do more complex work. I really enjoy the relationships I have with my patients, finding out about them and having a laugh with them.

**Sharon Jardine** @lindleydental

I love being a dentist because you can help someone go from being terrified of you and too ashamed to smile, to coming in to see you, grinning, proud of themselves and their smile.

**Pynadath George** @implantdude

Because it allows me to help others. Simple as that.

**Jaz Gulati** @jazzygulati

Not a single day is the same. If you really focus on the clinical scenario, there are nuances, complexities and challenges that are unique to each case. Even if you somehow get two identical clinical scenarios, they are attached to a person with emotions and values that will be different and require you to alter your management. Variety is the spice of life! That patient has put trust in you to manage the second most intimate area of their body. That's something special.

**Matt Parsons** @dr.matt.parsons

I really enjoyed dentistry from the first week of VT. I love having a laugh with colleagues in work, the environment and then taking this to my first patient and smiling with them.

**Hassan Maghaireh** @hassan_maghaireh
I love having the ability to be creative in offering my patients the wow experience in my own practice and growing that just as entrepreneurs grow their small businesses.

**Alfonso Rao** @dr.alfonso.rao
I really like to help people to get confidence back and I am still amazed every time that I see how people's personality can change when they are more confident with their smile or just simply happier to enjoy their food.

**Dipesh Kothari** @kothari.dental
I love the art, the people, the technology, the friendships, sharing knowledge and the never-ending quest for improvement. 'Perfection is a journey, not a destination.' - Someone clever.

**Sharron Parr** @lindleydental
I didn't know how to put into words why I love my job so much, but it came to me last week. When I write it down it seems too simple but it's people, I just love people. They come in all varieties (for want of a better word) and I love getting to know them and helping them.

**Mahrukh Khwaja** @mindninja.wellbeing
What I love the most about being a dentist is that every day we get the privilege to connect with our patients and help them in some way. Sometimes it's not even dental related, it's lending an ear during a divorce or cancer diagnosis or celebrating when they win. I love those moments and find that connection so meaningful.

**Riaz Yar** @riaz_yar_specialist

I love being a dentist because there is no other profession that encompasses art, engineering and physiology. It never bores as the patient is a complex jigsaw puzzle and getting to know them is a joy and challenge. This means I don't go to work. I go to learn.

**Simon Chard** @drsimonchard

I love the real human relationships I've built with my patients, the bond I have with some of these people will last a lifetime. I love that moment when the patient turns around the mirror and bursts into tears of happiness when they see their new smile. I love the combination of technology, art and biology working in and finally the dental community, it's great to have a community who all share a passion together.

**Ashley Latter** @ashley_latter

Many dentists have excellent technical skills, but have had very little training in communication skills. I have developed a programme that can really make a difference, allowing increased acceptance of treatment plans, allowing dentists to deliver the dentistry they love to do and their patients want. It's a win-win for everyone and that is why I have loved every minute of the last 25 years.

**Lukman Salaudeen** @lindleydental

I love being able to use my problem-solving skills and creativity to help bring satisfaction and better health to a wide range of people. Having to constantly learn and adapt means no two days are the same and this brings excitement to every day.

**Colin Campbell** @thecampbellacademy
I love being a dentist because it just fits my view of the world. It allows me to help people on a one-to-one basis when they're in trouble, but also to build something bigger and better and beyond me. It has allowed me to build a team that I am so proud of and a place that I feel the same way about. It has allowed me to travel on a journey, from being a 17-year-old boy to a 50-year-old man with amazing experiences, memories, friendships, and growth of learning. Dentistry has taken me to places that I could never have even imagined and has given me things beyond my wildest dreams.

**Marcos White** @marcoswhitedigital
I love being a dentist because it's given me an opportunity to express myself in creative and entrepreneurial ways. I enjoy the technical aspects and I love that we get to be with people, care for them and help them. I love it as a medium to be innovative and design new ways of doing things. I hope the things we've developed will leave a lasting impression on the profession.

**Chris Burton** @msgdental
I love being able to get into that 'zone', where I'm solving complex problems and doing fine work with my hands at the same time, all the while caring for and looking after the patient.

**Eimear O'Connell** @eimearkeenan22
I love the lifelong connection with our patients and the ability to change their dental destiny through education and teamwork.

**Aly Virani** @happyalyv

I love being a dentist because it is a career that has something for everyone. There is enough variety to find something that you enjoy, that challenges you, that allows you to help others and that pays your bills. And by bringing your personality to the table, your work can be an expression of yourself. Over time and with reflection and planning, I have truly found my happiness through dentistry. And I believe that everyone can.

**Ferhan Ahmed** @drferhanahmed

I love being a dentist because it allows me to make an impact and be creative every day.

**Kasia Allan** @katarzynaallan

In the early days when I was working as a dental nurse, I realised just how influential a beautiful smile and healthy teeth can be and just how neglected dentition can negatively impact our life. I'm passionate about dentistry. And also because we are privileged to help our patients and work with professionals that we can learn from and who will push us to take up new challenging opportunities.

**Toheed Hamid** @drhamidimplants

Dentistry allows me to intertwine science with art, creativity with academia, and passion with purpose. The gift of being able to use my skills to be at the service of others provides a lasting sense of fulfilment, and serves as an expression of gratitude for being blessed with those skills. Dentistry allows me to combine all this along with much more.

## Thomas Farrar @lindleydental

I love being a dentist because I get to use a fantastic mix of practical, intellectual and communication skills on a wide range of people from young children to the elderly. I especially enjoy getting people out of pain and find this very satisfying when they come back and they have none.

## Koray Feran @drkorayferan

It is one of those really worthwhile professions where you really get to make a difference to people's lives. It is a good mix of artistry and healthcare and I love the complexity of it. Being your own boss in a (generally) respected profession also counts for a lot and something we may take for granted.

## Matt Condon @mattcdentistry

I love the great relationships you can develop with patients, while helping to get them out of pain or improving their appearance. Getting to know them and their families is great, feels like being part of the community. Also getting to play with tools all day!

## Phil Reddington @philredbdt and Djemal Ibraimi @djemalibraimi

I'm not a painter, I'm not a sculptor or an artist, I'm not a CAD designer or CAM engineer, I'm not a photographer or a problem solver, I'm a dental technician. It pushes me to learn skills I never knew I had. Every case is different a new challenge, and to successfully negotiate through these cases and create teeth from wax, ceramic powders, plastics, gold, polymers, blocks of titanium and chrome I have had to apply all these skills. And that's why I love it!

### Tristan Tinn @tristanthedentist

I got into dentistry for the creativity, problem-solving, science, gadgets, fine motor skills, financial stability and relative flexibility. As I've grown as a clinician I've realised the importance of soft skills, communication and building relationships. This is what makes dentistry truly fulfilling, more than a perfectly blended margin ever will.

### Duncan Weir @dr.duncan_weir

I love being a dentist because you have complete freedom over your working hours, the variety of areas you can focus on and skills you can acquire. Every day is different and you get to help patients and people smile.

### Shaun Sellars @shaunsellars

For me, dentistry is more than just teeth. It's about the people that we meet on the way, the relationships we make and the lives that we affect. Every day of my working life there's one patient, or colleague, that makes the day worthwhile. And I know there'll be another one tomorrow. Dentistry isn't really about teeth. It's about people.

### Mark Topley @marktopley

I love working in dentistry. There are some great people doing brilliant work and it's been a privilege to provide them with opportunities to give back (when I was with Bridge2Aid) and have the opportunity to help them lead well (through my work now). Dentistry has given me a superb set of friends and fantastic experiences. I learn something new every day and work with talented, gifted and committed people.

**Kevin Armstrong** @denture.dude.uk
I love being a dental technician because we can work collaboratively with like minded professionals for successful outcomes for our patients.

**Pete Morris** petemorrisconsultancy.com
Anyone who provides a service has a responsibility to those who buy it. We don't just want people to make a financial transaction in our favour. We want them to come back to us because we want them to feel good. Entering into any service industry isn't about the profits or prestige. These things are hopeful outcomes. The reason we provide a service is because we believe we can make people's lives better as a result. That's our only purpose of our service.

**Ioan Rees** @drioanrees
If I had to single one great thing out about being a dentist is that you can get to a high level without wading through years of politics and sucking up to bosses. You're basically your own boss from a very early stage in your career and that's quite rare I think.

**Noel Perkins** @artistic.dental
I love being a dentist as I can be a doctor, an engineer, and an artist. Working as part of a team and being able to help patients by restoring their smile, ability to eat, self-confidence and quality of life makes this a fulfilling and fun career. I also have a passion for photography and dentistry allows me to explore and teach both documentary and artistic dental photography.

**Amit Mistry** @dramitmistry
I love being a dentist because it's an amazing career that allows you to do amazing things. If you can learn to do it properly, you can help so many people.

**Himesh Patel** @himeshpatel
I love being a dentist because the satisfaction one receives with the combination of high level technical skills, used to create artistry, to then transform someone's smile and confidence, is second to none!

**Paul Barnfather** @paul_wesleyan
I'm really proud of the work I do as a specialist adviser for dentists, but what really satisfies me the most is helping them to make their dreams come true and protecting what matters to them. The great relationships I have formed with my clients both on a professional and personal basis are what really make the job special.

**Robbie Williams** @dr.robbie.williams
I love the mix of skills and knowledge that dentistry demands of you; biology, art, physics, chemistry, mechanics, psychology and problem-solving. As a career, it challenges and rewards me in new ways every day, all while getting to help people and, on occasion, change their lives. I feel privileged to be able to do what I do.

**Louis Mackenzie** Head Dental Officer @denplan
Dentistry is an art-form based on scientific principles. Mastery of both the art and the science guarantees career-long rewards.

**Hazel Woodward** @lift__social
I love working within dentistry because I find it really empowering to see the changes dentists make to their patients. A few caring words are often all that's needed to allay a patient's nerves and anxiety, allowing them to access transformative treatments. Dentistry is a SUPERPOWER!

**Dhru Ratilal Shah** @dhru_soopercharger
The ability to influence behaviour change in a patient that could change their oral health for life - that's the magic. The ability to serve someone.

**John Lewis** @confidentalhelpline
I've not always been in love with dentistry but I look back now and remember the good times. The relationships I've built, the laughs I've had and the people I've helped, and I wouldn't change it for the world.

**Karl Walker-Finch** @drkarlsmiles
I love the blend of science, creativity and problem-solving skills that I use on a daily basis but for me, it's the people who are at the heart of it all. The patients of course, but also the wonderful teams I've been able to work with, the inspiring mentors, mentees and colleagues from across the globe.

# Acknowledgements

I am hugely grateful to all the dentists and students who gave their time to be interviewed when I was researching for this book. You have influenced a great many of these pages and I know the tapestry is much richer for each of your threads. I'd also like to thank everyone who contributed to the Why Do You Love Being in Dentistry? section. Your actions and words have inspired me and I know you will continue to inspire many more people for years to come.

A massive thank you to Vicky Quinn Fraser (@tinybeetlesteps) for the most epic book coaching, the constant reassurance kept me going and constructive feedback has made a world of difference. I'm proud to call myself a writer. Thank you also to Tee Twyford (@hustleandhush) for sharing her HUSTLE + hush process with me, I don't think I'd have been able to write this book without the way it changed how I use my energy and for letting me share that with the dental world. I owe a huge debt of gratitude to Hazel and Claire at Lift Social (@lift__social) for their marketing expertise and for getting the book launched in a way that people actually know about it.

I'm indebted to all my beta readers who provided priceless feedback, Daniel Eckford, David Hampson and Mark Foy, Chris Barrow, Thomas Farrar, Lukman Salaudeen, Christine Doherty and lastly Tristan Tinn who selflessly broke his wrist so he could have the time off to read the unedited shambles of a book in its entirety.

I'm eternally grateful to my Mum and Dad, for the beta reading, feedback and spell-checking, for supporting me when I told you I wanted to write a book at a time when you already thought I was too busy, but above all else, for being the best parents anyone could wish for.

Thank you to my kids who have brought so much joy and love into my life. You inspire me on a daily basis to live in the moment and to take joy in every minute we spend together.

Most of all, thank you to my incredible wife, Marisa, who has been a constant source of love and inspiration since the day we met. If it wasn't for you, not only would this book not have happened, I wouldn't be who I am today. Your direct contributions to this book are but a drop in the ocean compared to the influence you've had on my way of thinking and living. You smile, and then the spell was cast, and here we are in heaven, for you are mine, at last.

# Confidental

Confidental provide emotional first aid for dentists, hygienists, therapists and students in distress by lending an ear to talk to in complete confidence and when needed, signposting to further organisations. Often all we need is for someone to listen to us without judgement and Confidental offer that support.

The profits from the sales of this book are going to support the invaluable work they do at Confidental. If you've received a free copy of this book (please do pass this book on, don't let it gather dust on a shelf) then consider making a donation to them.

confidental-helpline.org

@confidentalhelpline

Tel: 0333 987 5158

# Marisa Walker-Finch

Marisa Walker-Finch is a BACP accredited psychotherapist who supports her clients with anxiety, depression, loss, stress and traumatic life events amongst many other things. With a foundation in person-centred therapy, she provides a blended approach for her clients including EMDR which has revolutionised the way she helps clients process trauma and overcome phobias.

Being married to a dentist, she has a unique insight into the challenges we can face in this profession. She provides most of her counselling online and so she can support her clients regardless of distance.

smilesintandem.com/counselling

Tel: 07538 798 025

# The Author

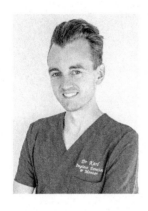

Karl Walker-Finch graduated from Liverpool Dental School in 2010. After nearly five years working on the Wirral, he moved with his wife Marisa to West Yorkshire where they started a family. Together they now own Smiles in Tandem, Huddersfield, a clinic that provides care for patients' dental and mental wellbeing in tandem.

Clinically, he spends the majority of his time providing dental implants and oral rehabilitation treatment on referral. Following his MSc in Dental Implantology with Distinction in 2017, he is now a senior mentor and lecturer on the master's programme at the University of Salford in association with ICE.

Karl is always looking for new opportunities to inspire others with his passion for dentistry on the subjects of dental implants, digital dentistry, mental wellbeing and personal development. On his website, you can access the resources mentioned in this book and find an extensive reading list that has inspired everything you've read.

WalkerFinch.com

@drkarlsmiles

Printed in Great Britain
by Amazon

35215100R00126